Power
Electronics

TUTORIAL GUIDES IN ELECTRONIC ENGINEERING

Series editors
Professor G.G. Bloodworth, *University of York*
Professor A.P. Dorey, *University of Lancaster*
Professor J.K. Fidler, *Open University*

This series is aimed at first- and second-year undergraduate courses. Each text is complete in itself, although linked with others in the series. Where possible, the trend towards a 'systems' approach is acknowledged, but classical fundamental areas of study have not been excluded. Worked examples feature prominently and indicate, where appropriate, a number of approaches to the same problem.

A format providing marginal notes has been adopted to allow the authors to include ideas and material to support the main text. These notes include references to standard mainstream texts and commentary on the applicability of solution methods, aimed particularly at covering points normally found difficult. Graded problems are provided at the end of each chapter, with answers at the end of the book.

Power Electronics

D.A. Bradley
Department of Engineering
University of Lancaster

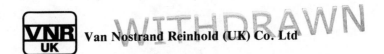 **VNR** **UK** **Van Nostrand Reinhold (UK) Co. Ltd**

First published in 1987 by
Van Nostrand Reinhold (UK) Co. Ltd
Molly Millars Lane, Wokingham, Berkshire, England

Reprinted 1987

Typeset in Times 10 on 12pt by
Colset Private Ltd, Singapore

Printed and bound in Hong Kong

British Library Cataloguing in Publication Data

Bradley, D.A.
    Power electronics. — (Tutorial guides in electronic engineering; 11).
    1. Electronics
    I. Title   II. Series
    537.5   TK7815

    ISBN 0-442-31778-6

ISSN 0266-2620

Contents

Preface

The subject of power electronics originated in the early part of the twentieth century with the development and application of devices such as the mercury arc rectifier and the thyratron valve. Indeed many of the circuits currently in use and described in this book were developed in that period. However, the range of applications for these early devices tended to be restricted by virtue of their size and problems of reliability and control.

With the development of power semiconductor devices, offering high reliability in a relatively compact form, power electronics began to expand its range and scope, with applications such as DC motor control and power supplies taking the lead. Initially, power semiconductor devices were available with only relatively low power levels and switching speeds. However, developments in device technology resulted in a rapid improvement in performance, accompanied by a corresponding increase in applications. These now range from power supplies using a single transistor to high voltage DC transmission where the mercury arc valve was replaced in the 1970s by a solid-state 'valve' using thyristor stacks.

Developments in microprocessor technology have also influenced the development of power electronics. This is particularly apparent in the areas of control, where analogue controllers are being replaced by digital systems, and in the evolution of the 'smart power' devices. These developments have in turn led to system improvements in areas such as robot drives, power supplies and railway traction systems.

To a professional engineer, power electronics encompasses all of the above, from the mercury arc rectifier systems still operational to the microprocessor-controlled drives on a robot arm. However, to deal with all of these topics is outside the scope of this book which therefore concentrates on providing the reader with an introduction to the subject of power electronics. Following a discussion of the major power electronic devices and their characteristics, with relatively little consideration given to device physics, the emphasis is placed on the systems aspects of power electronics and on the range and diversity of applications. For this reason, a number of 'mini case studies' are included in the chapters on applications. These case studies cover topics from high-voltage DC transmission to the development of a controller for domestic appliances such as washing machines and are intended to place the material under discussion into a practical context.

As the text is intended for instruction and learning rather than for reference, each chapter includes a number of worked examples for emphasis and reinforcement. These worked examples are supported further by a number of exercises at the end of each chapter.

The production of a book of this type does not proceed in isolation and many people have contributed to it, either by the provision of material or with encouragement and advice. From among my colleagues at Lancaster University I would particularly thank Professor Tony Dorey, who encouraged me to undertake the project and provided much helpful advice, and David Dawson for reading and commenting on certain of the material. Elsewhere, Dr. Peter White of Plymouth

Polytechnic provided valuable assistance through his comments on the early drafts.

As this book is one of a series of related texts, its relationship with the other texts in the series is important. I am therefore grateful to Professor John Sparkes of the Open University for his help in this respect, particularly with Chapter 1.

I would also thank Mr. A. Woodworth of Mullard, Mr. J.M.W. Whiting of GEC Traction, Mr I.E. Barker of GEC Power Transmission and Distribution Projects, Mr. T.G. Carthy of Renold plc, Mr. A. Polkinghorne of Polkinghorne Industries and Dr. P. McEwan, all of whom helped with the provision of material.

As the book is intended for students, a student's viewpoint at an early stage proved particularly valuable and I would thank Michael Anson for diverting himself from his studies to help me in that respect. Finally, but by no means least, my thanks to my Consulting Editor, Professor G. Bloodworth of York University for his efforts, constructive comments and assistance in this project.

Power Semiconductors

☐ To introduce the major power electronic devices.
☐ To define their operating regimes and modes of operation.
☐ To establish their ratings.
☐ To consider losses and heat transfer properties.
☐ To examine means of protection.

An intrinsic semiconductor is defined as being a material having a resistivity which lies between that of insulators and conductors and which decreases with increasing temperature. The principal semiconductor material used for power electronic devices is silicon, a member of Group IV of the periodic table of elements which means it has four electrons in its outer orbit.

If an element of Group V, such as phosphorus, with five electrons in its outer orbit is added to the silicon, each phosphorus atom forms a covalent bond within the silicon lattice, leaving a loosely bound electron. The presence of these additional electrons greatly increases the conductivity of the silicon and a material doped in this way is referred to as an n-type semiconductor.

By introducing an element from Group III as impurity, a vacant bonding location or hole is introduced into the lattice. This hole may be considered to be mobile as it can be filled by an adjacent electron, which in its turn leaves a hole behind. Holes can be thought of as carriers of positive charge and a semiconductor doped by a Group III impurity is referred to as a p-type semiconductor.

The extra, mobile electrons introduced by doping into the n-type material and the equivalent holes in the p-type material are referred to as the majority carriers. In an n-type material there is a small population of holes and in a p-type material a small population of electrons. These are called the minority carriers.

Diode

The semiconductor junction diode shown in Fig. 1.1 is the simplest semiconductor device used in power electronics. With no external applied voltage the redistribution of charges in the region of the junction between the p-type and n-type materials results in an equilibrium condition in which a potential barrier is established across a narrow region depleted of charge carriers on each side of the junction. This equilibrium may be disturbed by the application of an external applied voltage of either polarity.

If a reverse voltage — cathode positive with respect to anode — is applied, the electric field at the junction is reinforced, increasing the height of the potential

Ghandi, S.K. (1977). *Semiconductor Power Devices*. Wiley Interscience.

Sparkes, J. *Semiconductor Devices*. (1987). Van Nostrand Reinhold.

The region over which the potential barrier exists is known as the depletion or transition layer.

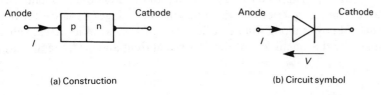

(a) Construction (b) Circuit symbol

Fig. 1.1   The diode.

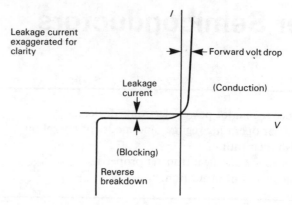

Fig. 1.2 Diagrammatic representation of the diode static characteristic. [Note: Forward and reverse voltage scales are unequal. The forward voltage drop is of the order of 1 V while the reverse breakdown voltage varies from a few 10 s of volts to several thousand volts.]

The magnitude of the reverse leakage current can vary from a few picoamperes for an integrated circuit diode to a few milliamperes for a power diode capable of carrying several thousand amperes in the forward direction.

Avalanche diodes are designed to operate safely under reverse breakdown conditions and are used for device overvoltage protection. See section on protection, Chapter 1.

barrier and increasing the energy required by a majority carrier to cross this barrier. The resulting small reverse leakage current shown in the diode static characteristic of Fig. 1.2 is due to the flow of minority carriers across the junction. The magnitude of the reverse leakage current increases with temperature because the number of minority carriers available increases with the temperature of the material.

The reverse current will be maintained with increasing reverse voltage up to the point at which reverse breakdown occurs, which will not cause the destruction of the diode unless accompanied by excessive heat generation.

When a forward voltage — anode positive with respect to cathode — is applied to the diode the height of the potential barrier is reduced, giving rise to a forward current resulting from the flow of majority carriers across the junction. As the forward voltage is increased, the forward current through the diode increases exponentially. The overall current–voltage characteristic of the diode is given approximately by

$$I = I_s[\exp(qV_j/kT) - 1]$$ (1.1)

where I_s is the reverse leakage current
q is the electronic charge (1.602×10^{-19} C)
k is Boltzmann's constant (1.38×10^{-23} J/K)
V_j is the voltage applied to the junction
and T is the temperature (K)

giving the forward or conducting part of the diode characteristic of Fig. 1.2. The forward voltage (V_j) applied to the junction is of the order of 0.7 V but because of internal resistances in series with the junction, the voltage (V) across the terminals of a practical power diode will be of the order of 1 V, with the actual value being determined by the magnitude of the forward current and device temperature.

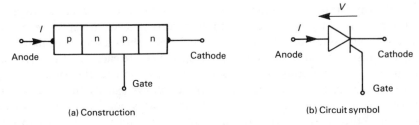

(a) Construction   (b) Circuit symbol

Fig. 1.3 The thyristor.

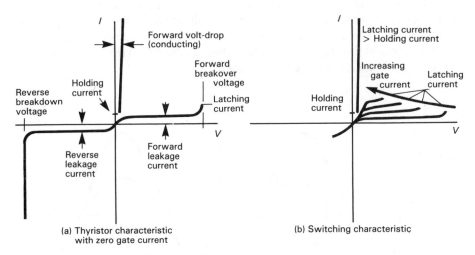

(a) Thyristor characteristic with zero gate current   (b) Switching characteristic

Fig. 1.4 Thyristor characteristics.

Thyristor

The thyristor is a four-layer, three-terminal device as shown in Fig. 1.3. The three p–n junctions of the thyristor are so close together that they interact in a manner which is too complex to be explained here. However, in order to be able to use the thyristor it is necessary to understand both its behaviour as a circuit element and its characteristics.

The static characteristic of a thyristor with no gate current applied is shown by Fig. 1.4(a). With a reverse voltage applied the characteristic is similar to that of a diode with a small reverse leakage current flowing up to the point of reverse breakdown. When a forward voltage is applied a forward leakage current will flow, rising to the latching current level at the forward breakover voltage. Following forward breakover, the two central regions of the thyristor are flooded with holes and electrons, forward biasing the central junction to turn the thyristor ON. The forward voltage drop then falls to a value between 1 V and 2 V.

The thyristor can also be switched to the ON or conducting state by injecting a current into the central p-type layer via the gate terminal. The injection of the gate current provides additional holes in the central p-type layer, reducing the forward breakover voltage to a value less than the applied voltage and turning the thyristor ON. These conditions are illustrated in Fig. 1.4(b), showing the effect of increasing gate current on the level of forward breakover voltage.

Silicon Controlled Rectifier Manual. General Electric, (1979). New York.

Power Semiconductor Handbook. Semikron, (1980).

Blicher, A. (1976). *Thyristor Physics*. Springer-Verlag.

The forward breakover and reverse breakdown voltages for a thyristor are approximately equal in magnitude.

Once the thyristor has been turned on it will continue to conduct as long as the forward current remains above the holding current level, irrespective of gate current or circuit conditions. Figures 1.5(a) and 1.5(b) show a single, ideal thyristor supplying a resistive and an inductive load respectively. In each case the thyristor is being turned on after a delay of about a quarter of a cycle after the voltage zero. In the case of the resistive load the load current follows exactly the load voltage. However, in the case of the inductive load the load voltage is made up of two components, the voltage across the inductance (v_i) and the voltage across the resistance (v_r) and the current through the thyristor has an initial value of zero. The current then rises to a maximum at which point di/dt and hence the voltage across the inductance (v_i) becomes zero and the load voltage (v_L) equals the voltage across the resistor (v_r). The slope of di/dt then becomes negative, changing the polarity of v_i, and thus maintains the forward voltage drop across the thyristor until the stored energy in the inductance has been dissipated.

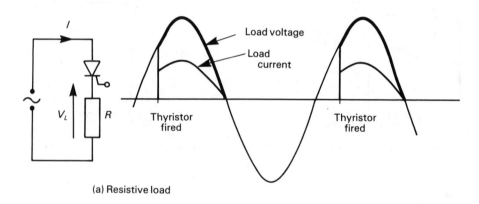

(a) Resistive load

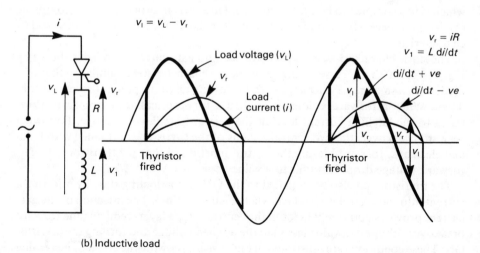

(b) Inductive load

Fig. 1.5   Thyristor with different loads.

Turn-on

Following the initiation of forward breakover by the gate current the process of establishing conduction is independent of the gate conditions once the thyristor current has reached the latching current level. The time taken for the thyristor current to reach the latching current level therefore establishes the minimum period over which the gate current must be maintained.

The time interval between the application of the gate current and the point at which the thyristor current reaches 90% of its final value is referred to as the *turn-on time*. This time is made up of two components, the *delay time*, which is the time taken for the current to reach 10% of its final value, and the *rise time*, which is the time for the current to increase from 10% to 90% of its final value. The relationship between these values is illustrated by Fig. 1.6. The rate of rise of current in the thyristor is influenced by the load inductance, with increasing inductance extending the turn-on time.

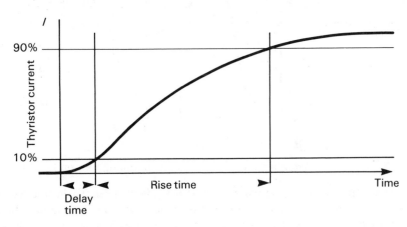

Fig. 1.6   Thyristor current on turn-on.

A thyristor with a latching current of 40 mA is used in the circuit shown. If a firing pulse of 50 μs is applied at the instant of maximum source voltage, show that the thyristor will not be turned on. What value of resistance R' connected as shown will ensure turn-on?

Worked Example 1.1

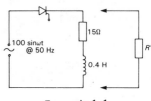

Example 1.1

Following the application of the gate pulse

$100 \cos \omega t = iR + L di/dt$

Using Laplace Transforms

$i = 100 [\cos(\omega t - \phi) - \cos\phi. \exp(-Rt/L)]/(R^2 + \omega^2 L^2)^{1/2}$

$\phi = \tan^{-1}\omega L/R = 83.19° = 1.452$ rad

$(R^2 + \omega^2 L^2)^{1/2} = 126.6$

After 50 μs, by substituting in equation for i

$i = 0.0124$ A

Hence thyristor fails to turn on.

Connecting R' then current in R' is i' when

Current in thyristor = $i_t = i + i'$

For turn-on

$$i + i' = 0.04 \text{ A}$$
$$\therefore \quad i' = 40 - 12.4 = 27.6 \text{ mA}$$

Maximum value of R' is thus

$$100 \cos (100 \, \pi \times 50 \times 10^{-6})/0.0276 = 3623 \, \Omega$$

The turn-on time will also be limited by the need to avoid conditions of high rate of rise of current at high forward voltage levels as the instantaneous product of current and voltage (power) can be high, resulting in damage to the thyristor by thermal effects. Figure 1.7 shows a typical power relationship for a 150 A thyristor.

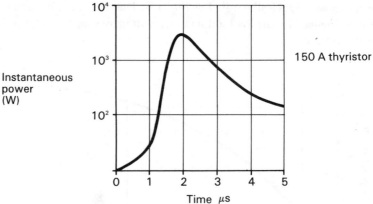

Fig. 1.7   Instantaneous power in thyristor during turn-on.

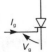

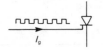

The gate signal required to turn on a thyristor is influenced by the gate voltage versus gate current relationship for the particular thyristor. The actual characteristic for a given type of thyristor will lie between the definable limits of the gate high resistance and gate low resistance lines of Fig. 1.8. Further constraints are placed on the gate signal by the limiting values of gate current, gate voltage, gate power and temperature. Combining these limits gives the full gate characteristic of Fig. 1.8.

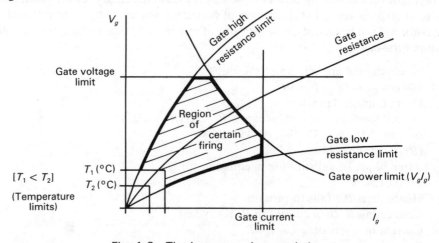

Fig. 1.8   Thyristor gate characteristic.

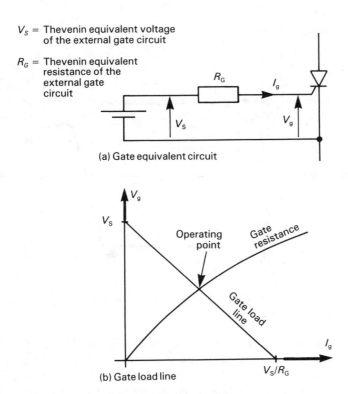

V_S = Thevenin equivalent voltage of the external gate circuit

R_G = Thevenin equivalent resistance of the external gate circuit

(a) Gate equivalent circuit

(b) Gate load line

Fig. 1.9   Gate operation.

The actual operating point is obtained from consideration of the circuit of Fig. 1.9. This circuit defines the gate load line (slope $= -R_G$), the intersection of which with the thyristor gate resistance characteristic determines the gate operating point.

Typically, thyristor firing circuits use pulse techniques which allow a precise control of the point-on-wave at which the thyristor is fired and which dissipate less energy in the gate than a continuous current. Reliance is not usually placed on a single pulse to fire the thyristor but instead the firing circuit is arranged to generate a train of pulses.

Reverse voltage, cathode positive with respect to the anode.

Turn-off

Turn-off of a thyristor begins when the forward current falls below the holding current level of Fig. 1.4(a) with no gate current applied. Turn-off performance depends on device characteristics, the forward current prior to turn-off, the peak reverse current and the rate of rise of forward voltage as well as temperature effects. Once the current has fallen to zero the thyristor must be placed into the reverse blocking state with a reverse voltage applied across the thyristor for sufficient time to allow the potential barriers to be re-established, completing the turn-off.

See Chapter 3 for details of forced commutation circuits.

The dynamic behaviour of the thyristor during turn-off is shown in Fig. 1.10. Initially, the forward current falls, reaching zero at time t_0 and then reverses. From t_0 to t_1 the reverse current is sustained by the large numbers of carriers previously

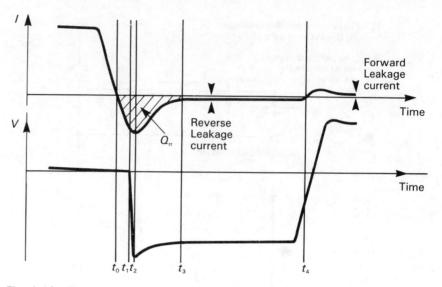

Fig. 1.10   Thyristor current and voltage during turn-off with zero gate current.

injected into the thyristor and device voltage drop is small. The build-up of the potential barriers at the junctions between and the removal of charge carriers by the action of the reverse current in the interval from t_1 to t_2 means that at time t_2 the reverse current can no longer be sustained and it begins to reduce. At this point the full reverse voltage appears across the junction, and as the circuit is slightly inductive this voltage will overshoot slightly, driving the reverse current down to the level of the reverse leakage current.

The carrier stored charge recovered during this period is shown as the shaded area of Fig. 1.10 and is referred to as the *reverse recovery charge* (Q_{rr}). Although the reverse recovery period is completed at time t_3, the reverse voltage must be maintained until time t_4 to ensure that the carrier density in the region of the central junction is reduced to a sufficiently small level to prevent the possibility of turn-on occuring when a forward voltage is reapplied. The total time for turn-off will vary according to the thyristor but will typically lie in the range 10 to 100 μs.

This occurs with all p–n junctions when changing from a forward biased to a reverse biased condition. Sparkes, J. *Semiconductor Devices* (1987). Van Nostrand Reinhold.

These conditions for turn-off occur automatically in a naturally commutated converter such as those described in Chapter 2. There is, however, a range of circuits operating from a DC voltage source in which additional circuitry must be used to turn the thyristor off. These additional, forced commutation circuits first force a reverse current through the thyristor for a short time to reduce the forward current to zero and then maintain the reverse voltage for the necessary time interval to complete the turn-off.

See Chapter 3 for details of forced commutation circuits.

Parallel and series operation of thyristors

To accommodate high load currents a parallel connection of thyristors can be used. If the simple connection of Fig. 1.11(a) is used then differences in the individual thyristors will result in an unequal sharing of current between them. This sharing can be evened out by the careful selection of matched devices, by the use of series resistance, as in Fig. 1.11(b), or by including current-sharing reactors as in Fig. 1.11(c).

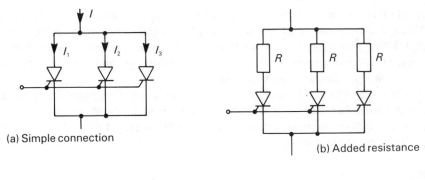

(a) Simple connection

(b) Added resistance

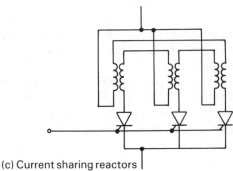

(c) Current sharing reactors

Fig. 1.11　Parallel connection of thyristors.

At turn-on the thyristor gate circuits must all be hard driven from the same source to force a simultaneous turn-on of all devices. To prevent any individual thyristor from turning off if its current falls below its holding level a continuous gate signal is normally used to ensure immediate re-firing.

Where high voltage levels are encountered thyristors can be connected in series to share the voltage. If the connection of Fig. 1.12(a) is used then the differences between the individual devices can result in an unequal voltage sharing between them. Allowance must also be made for any difference in recovery times to ensure

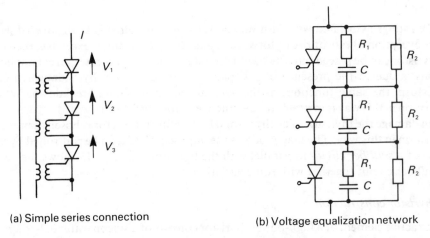

(a) Simple series connection

(b) Voltage equalization network

Fig. 1.12　Series connection of thyristors.

that all thyristors are left able to withstand the reapplication of forward voltage.

Voltage sharing can be achieved by using equalization networks such as that of Fig. 1.12(b). The capacitors ensure that each thyristor recovers fully on turn-off, while the resistor R_1 prevents an excessive di/dt on turn-on and resistor R_2 provides for equal steady-state sharing of voltage.

As the gates of the individual thyristors can be separated by potentials of several thousand volts and gate pulse must be provided from a common source via some means of isolation such as transformers, optically coupled diodes or transistors and fibre-optic light guides.

Gate circuit isolation.

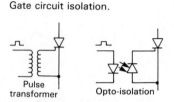

Pulse transformer   Opto-isolation

See Chapter 5, case study of the Cross-Channel HVDC link.

Ratings

Operation of a thyristor is limited by the various ratings which define the operating boundaries. These ratings include the peak, average and RMS currents, the peak forward and reverse voltages and the gate circuit limits. In addition there are several transient limits to be considered.

Short-duration overloads will result in an increase in the internal temperature of the thyristor with little outward heat transfer. Taking the device internal losses to be proportional to the square of the current, the internal temperature rise can be expressed by an $\int i^2 dt$ value. Thyristors are therefore given an $\int i^2 dt$ rating which relates to the maximum permitted temperature rise.

Worked Example 1.2

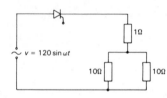

$v = 120 \sin \omega t$

A thyristor has an $\int i^2 dt$ rating of 15 amp²s and is being used to supply the circuit shown from a 120 V AC supply when a fault occurs, short-circuiting the 10 Ω resistors to earth. What is the shortest fault clearance time to be achieved if damage to the thyristor is to be prevented?

Worst-case fault occurs when voltage is at maximum. Assume that the voltage is at its maximum value for the duration of the fault, then

$$\int_0^{t_c} i^2 dt = \int_0^{t_c} 120^2 \, dt = 15$$

∴   Fault clearance time $= 15/120^2 = 1.04$ ms

The ratings associated with turn-on and turn-off have already been covered with the exception of rate of rise of forward voltage (dV/dt). If this is excessive, then the thyristor can be placed into the conducting state even with no gate current applied. This is due to the presence of a capacitive current in the thyristor which can perform the same functions as the gate current in initiating breakdown. While turn-on in this way is in itself non-destructive of the thyristor, repeated occurrences can damage the thyristor. The thyristor dV/dt rating is therefore chosen to prevent turn-on in this way. The magnitude of the imposed dV/dt can be controlled by the use of a *snubber circuit* in parallel with the thyristor. Figure 1.13 shows the basic snubber circuit together with some variations.

See section on Protection, Chapter 1 for the use of voltage controlled resistors, avalanche diodes and selenium rectifiers for device protection.

Thyristor construction

The active element of a high-power thyristor consists of a silicon wafer 0.2–0.3 mm thick and with a diameter up to 80 mm or more. This wafer must be carried in a

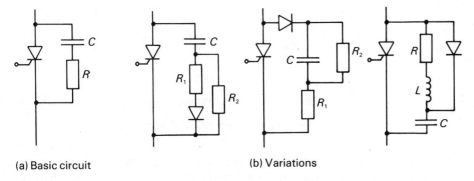

(a) Basic circuit   (b) Variations

Fig. 1.13 Snubber circuits.

housing designed to provide the necessary connections to the anode, cathode and gate as well as being mechanically robust to allow the thyristor to he handled with safety. It must also have suitable heat transfer properties for the purpose of device cooling.

The principal constructions used for thyristors are the stud-base, capsule and for lower-power applications the flat pack assemblies shown in Fig. 1.14.

Gate Turn-Off Thyristor

The gate turn-off (GTO) thyristor, the symbol for which is shown in Fig. 1.15(a), is a variant of the thyristor in which the internal structure has been modified to enable

Taylor, P.D. (1984). GTO thyristor device design. *Electronics and Power*, 463–6.

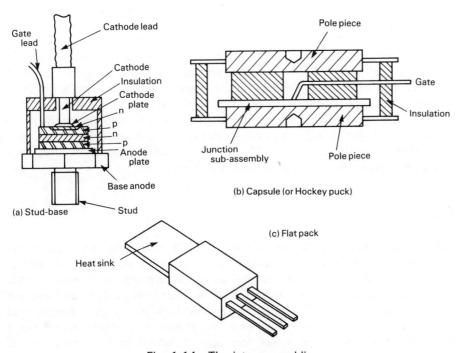

(a) Stud-base

(b) Capsule (or Hockey puck)

(c) Flat pack

Fig. 1.14 Thyristor assemblies.

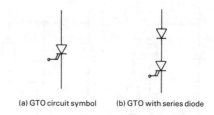

(a) GTO circuit symbol   (b) GTO with series diode

Fig. 1.15   Gate turn-off (GTO) thyristor.

Burgum, F.J. (1982). The GTO — a new power switch. *Electronics and Power*, 389–92.

See Chapter 3.

Williams, B.W. and Palmer, P.R. (1984). Drive and snubber circuits for GTOs and power transistors — particularly for inverter bridges. IEE Conference Publication 234, *Power Electronics and Variable Speed Drives*, 42–5.

Hall, J.K. and Manning, C.D. (1984). Switching properties of GTO thyristors. IEE Conference Publication 234, *Power Electronics and Variable Speed Drives*, 958–61.

Woodworth, A. (1981). Understanding GTO data as an aid to circuit design. *Electronic Components and Applications* 3(3).

Asymmetric thyristor.

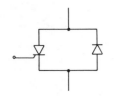

Triac firing. Typically a negative gate current would be used to initiate both forward and reverse conduction.

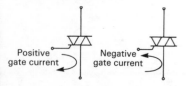

Positive gate current   Negative gate current

the forward current to be turned off by the application of a negative gate current. Though the GTO thyristor was a relatively early development in thyristor technology, the limitations on its operating power levels and developments in power transistors, meant that it found little application initially. More recently, developments in both device technology and control systems, particularly those employing microprocessors, has led to a growth in GTO applications, particularly in pulse-width modulated inverter drives.

On turn-on, the GTO thyristor must be supplied with a high initial gate current to establish the conduction. Then, unlike the conventional thyristor where the gate signal may be removed once conduction is established, the gate current of the GTO thyristor must be maintained at the level necessary to prevent any possible drop-out from the conducting state. On turn-off the current must be rapidly diverted from the gate of the GTO to ensure a rapid and effective turn-off.

A limitation of the GTO thyristor is its reduced reverse breakdown voltage in relation to a conventional thyristor. To accommodate this, a series diode may need to be included, as in Fig. 1.15(b).

Asymmetric Thyristor

The asymmetric thyristor is a combination of a thyristor and a reverse diode in parallel on the same wafer. It is therefore controllable in the thyristor forward direction and will always conduct in the reverse direction. The asymmetric thyristor finds applications in circuits such as inverters where an inverse parallel diode is often employed in conjunction with a thyristor to accomodate the phase shift of current with an inductive load. By incorporating both devices on the same wafer they are in the closest possible proximity, reducing effects such as stray inductance which may otherwise influence performance.

Triac

The triac is a multilayer device that is electrically the same as two thyristors connected in inverse parallel on the same wafer. Figure 1.16 shows the make up of a triac together with its circuit symbol and static characteristic. As the terms anode and cathode have no real meaning for triacs, the terms *terminal 1* (T_1) and *terminal 2* (T_2) are used. The gate signal is then applied between the gate terminal and terminal 1. The triac can be turned on by the injection of either a positive or a negative gate current. It is, however, most sensitive when a positive gate current is used with terminal 2 at a positive potential (forward conduction) or a negative gate

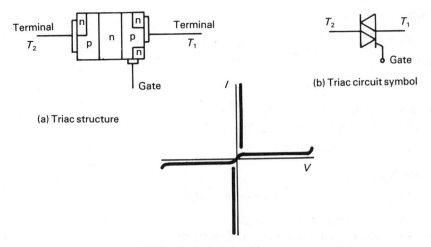

(a) Triac structure

(b) Triac circuit symbol

(c) Triac characteristic with zero gate current

Fig. 1.16   The triac.

current with terminal 1 at a positive potential (reverse conduction). The least sensitive condition is a positive gate current applied with terminal 1 at a positive potential.

A derivative of the triac is the *diac*. This is a gateless triac arranged to break down at a low voltage in both the forward and reverse directions. It is used in trigger circuits such as that of Fig. 1.17 where variation of the resistance varies the phase angle of the diac voltage with respect to the supply voltage and hence controls the point-on-wave at which the diac breakdown voltage is reached, varying the firing point of the triac.

Diac circuit symbol and characteristic.

Diac

Worked Example 1.3

A diac with a breakdown voltage of 40 V is used in a circuit such as that of Fig. 1.17, with R_1 variable from 1000 to 25 000 Ω, $C = 470$ nF, and $V = 240$ V RMS at 50 Hz.

What will be the maximum and minimum firing delays with this arrangement?

Impedance of capacitor $= 1/\omega C = 6773 \ \Omega = |Z_c|$

The current through R_1 and C when the diac is not conducting is

$$i_d = 240 \sqrt{2} \sin(\omega t + \phi)/Z_d$$

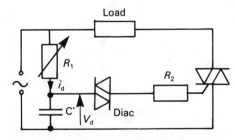

Fig. 1.17   Triac firing circuit using a diac.

where

$$Z_d = (R_1{}^2 + 1/\omega^2C^2)^{1/2}$$

and

$$\phi = \tan^{-1}(1/\omega RC)$$

With $R_1 = 1000\ \Omega$, $Z_d = 6846\ \Omega$
The voltage across the capacitor is $i_d Z_c = v_c$

$$v_c = 335.8\sin(\omega t - 8.4°)$$

When diac conducts, $v_c = 40$ V

$\therefore$ Minimum delay $= \sin^{-1}(40/335.8) + 8.4° = 15.24°$

With $R_1 = 25\,000\ \Omega$, $Z_d = 25\,901\ \Omega$
The voltage across the capacitor is $i_d Z_c$ as before

$$v_c = 88.76\sin(\omega t - 74.84°)$$

When diac conducts, $v_c = 40$ V
Hence

$$\text{Maximum delay} = \sin^{-1}(40/88.76) + 74.84° = 101.6°$$

Power Transistor

Blicher, A. (1981). *Field-effect and Bipolar Power Transistor Physics.* Academic Press.

This device is known as a bipolar transistor as both holes and electrons are active.

The base emitter junction can fail at voltages of the order of 10 V.

The transistor is a three-layer, semiconductor device as shown in Fig. 1.18(a) and has the characteristic of Fig. 1.19(a). Forward breakdown occurs with increasing collector–emitter voltage (V_{CE}) in a fashion similar to the previous devices. However, reverse breakdown of the base–emitter junction takes place at a relatively low voltage level. A series diode is therefore used as in Fig. 1.20 to protect against the reversal of V_{CE}.

Conventionally, the transistor is used as an amplifier when:

$$I_C = \beta I_B$$

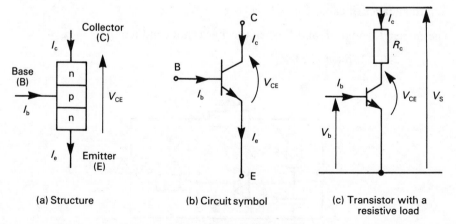

(a) Structure   (b) Circuit symbol   (c) Transistor with a resistive load

Fig. 1.18 NPN power transistor.

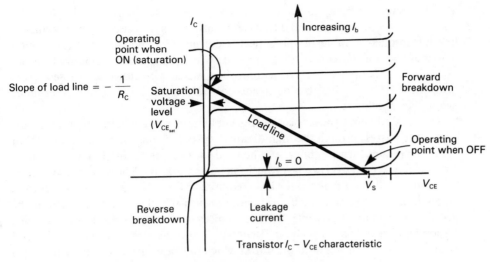

Fig. 1.19a   Transistor characteristics [Note: forward and reverse voltage scales are unequal.]

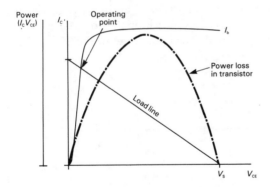

Fig. 1.19b   Variation in power loss in a transistor with variation in V_{CE} constant load R_C.

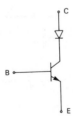

Fig. 1.20   Transistor with series diode.

For a transistor operating with a resistive load as in Fig. 1.18(c), operation is constrained to follow the load line shown on Fig. 1.19(a) since:

$$I_C = (V_s - V_{CE})/R_c \qquad (1.2)$$

As I_B is increased from 0 to the value required to drive the transistor into saturation

15

$V_{CE,sat} \simeq 1.1 \text{ V}.$

the collector current increases and V_{CE} decreases correspondingly. The instantaneous power loss in the transistor during this transition is the product of the instantaneous value of the collector current (I_C) and the collector–emitter voltage (V_{CE}) and varies according to Fig. 1.19(b). In power electronic applications the transistor is used entirely as a controlled switch with either zero base current (transistor OFF) or in saturation (transistor ON), as the losses in any other mode would be prohibitive.

The losses in the transistor due to switching can nevertheless be high as the transistor passes through the high dissipation state during each transition ON or OFF. To reduce turn-on times, and hence device power dissipation, a high initial base current is used to give a fast transition into saturation. The base current is then reduced to and maintained at the level required to keep the transistor in saturation to minimize the losses in the base circuit. On turn-off, the base current should be reduced as rapidly as possible. There is, however, a complex phenomenon called 'secondary breakdown' which can occur with fast transients, resulting in failure of the transistor which will limit the rate at which the base current can be reduced. In order to improve turn-off a reverse base current is applied to the transistor and a reverse bias maintained in the off condition.

The safe operating region (SOAR) of the transistor, shown in Fig. 1.21, defines the safe limits of operation in terms of I_c and V_{CE}. For safe operation the instantaneous values of I_c and V_{CE} must lie within the boundaries of this curve at all times within the switching interval. The boundaries of the SOAR are adjusted as shown on the figure to take account of single-pulse operation, with pulses of varying duration.

Darlington base-drive circuit.

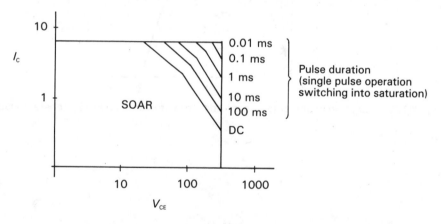

Basic Darlington circuit

Practical Darlington circuit

Fig. 1.21   Transistor safe operating region.

Though the transistor can switch more rapidly than the thyristor, times of a few microseconds being achievable, the need to supply a base current to maintain it in the ON condition means that the requirements of the base drive circuit are more severe than those of the thyristor gate circuit. Typically, a thyristor will require a pulse of a few milliamperes lasting for a few microseconds to turn it on while an equivalently rated transistor will require a continuous base current, possibly of several amperes, to keep it turned on.

Some power transistors incorporate a base drive circuit on the same chip as the

main power transistor. This arrangement reduces the external base current requirements but at the cost of some increase in switching time.

A transistor has the switching characteristic shown in the figures. If the mean
power loss in the transistor is limited to 200 W, what is the maximum switching rate
that can be achieved?

Worked Example 1.4

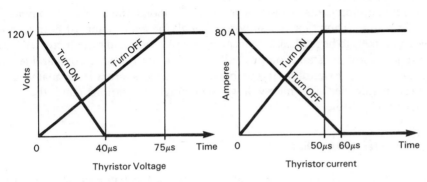

Example 1.4

Energy loss in transistor = $\displaystyle\int_0^t i_c V_{CE}\, dt$

Turn-on energy loss = $\displaystyle\int_0^{40\times10^{-6}} 120(1 - 2.5 \times 10^4 t) \times 1.6 \times 10^6 t\, dt = 51\ \text{mJ}$

Turn-off energy loss = $\displaystyle\int_0^{60\times10^{-6}} 1.6 \times 10^6 t \times 80(1 - 1.667 \times 10^4 t)\, dt = 76.8\ \text{mJ}$

Total loss in one cycle = 127.8 mJ
Number of cycles in one second = 200/0.1278 = 1564.9

Power MOS

Increasing demands for higher-frequency operation of power electronics devices
for applications such as the switched mode power supply has led to the development of power MOSFETs. These operate with low switching losses and require
much lower levels of gate current than the base current of the equivalent rated
transistor to maintain them in the ON condition. This low gate current requirement
means that it is often possible to drive a power MOS device directly from standard
logic, LSI circuit output and microcomputer ports. As the gate circuit is largely
capacitive the gate current source must be properly matched, particularly where
high-speed operation is required.

At lower voltage levels the ON resistance of a power MOSFET tends to be less
than that of the equivalent transistor, lying in the range 0.05–0.25 Ω for a 100 V
device and 2–8 Ω for a 1000 V device. This resistance increases with the voltage
across the device (V_{DS}) according to $V_{DS}^{2.6}$ and with junction temperature, with an
approximate doubling between 25°C and 125°C for a higher voltage device. This

See Chapter 5.

MOS *M*etal *O*xide
*S*emiconductor; FET *F*ield *E*ffect
*T*ransistor.

Reid, J. (1982). The power
MOSFET — a user's view.
Electronics and Power, 393–5.

MOSFET construction (see also reference 1.2).

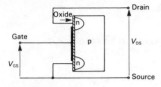

Foster, A. (1984). Trends in power semiconductors. IEE Conf. Pub. 234, *Power Electronics and Variable Speed Drives*, 1–6.

The ambient temperature heat sink is taken as being a constant-temperature system whose temperature is not altered by any additional energy input.

means that at higher voltages MOSFETs tend to be limited to lower currents than transistors or thyristors of similar voltage rating. The application of power MOS devices is also restricted by the fact that the technology used in their manufacture is currently more expensive than that required for the production of the other main power electronics devices.

Therefore, though lower voltage power MOS devices are price competitive, at higher voltage levels some system advantage such as high switching rates will normally be required to justify their use.

Current developments include the merging of bipolar and MOS technologies on a single crystal. Though a system possessing all the good points of both technologies is unlikely to be realizable, such devices typically would offer increased input sensitivity, a low resistance output and switching performance comparable with bipolar devices. Examples of combinational devices are the Insulated Gate Transistor intended for high-voltage switching applications, and the Static Induction Thyristor.

Heat Transfer and Cooling

The heat generated in a power semiconductor device due to internal losses has to be conducted away from the device and dissipated. In a thyristor, the internal heat source is taken to be a junction within the semiconductor material. The heat transfer path is then:

(1) from the junction to the case of the device;
(2) from the casing to a heat transfer system such as a fin;
(3) from the heat transfer system to the final ambient temperature heat sink.

The effect of the different thermal characteristics of these various stages in the heat removal process is analogous to a chain of resistors and capacitors fed from a current source. An equivalent circuit describing the thermal performance can therefore be formed using thermal resistance and capacitance as in Fig. 1.22.

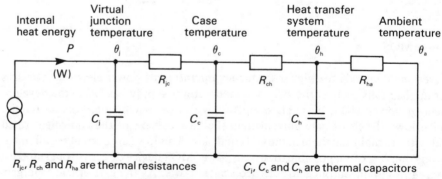

Fig. 1.22   Heat transfer path.

Temperature differences are analogous to voltage differences and heat flow is analogous to current flow. This leads to an analogy between electrical and thermal components:

Electrical		*Thermal*	
Charge	$C = As$	Heat	$J = Ws$

Current	A		Heat flow	W	
Potential difference	V		Temperature difference	°C	
Resistance	V/A		Thermal resistance	°C/W	
Capacitance	As/V		Thermal capacitance	Ws/°C	

Under steady-state conditions the thermal capacitance has no effect and the heat flow out of the device can be represented by the series combination of the thermal resistances.

$$\theta_j = \theta_a + P(R_{jc} + R_{ch} + R_{ha}) \qquad (1.3)$$

Thermal analogue of Ohm's Law. Thermal resistance R = (Temperature difference)/(Power transferred) = $(\theta_1 - \theta_2)/P$ (°C/W).

where θ_j = Temperature of the junction (°C)
  θ_a = Ambient temperature (°C)
  P = Internal power loss (W)
  R_{jc} = Thermal resistance, junction to casing (°C/W)
  R_{ch} = Thermal resistance, casing to heat transfer system (°C/W)
  R_{ha} = Thermal resistance, heat transfer system to heat sink (°C/W).

The effect of using forced or liquid cooling is to increase the rate of heat removal, reducing R_{ha}.

A thyristor has a thermal resistance of 0.82°C/W between its virtual junction and the heat transfer system and 1.96°C/W between the heat transfer system and the ambient temperature heat sink. What will be the power loss in the thyristor if the junction temperature is to be kept below 132°C for an ambient temperature of 28°C?

Worked Example 1.5

From Equation 1.2,

$$132 = 28 + P(0.82 + 1.96)$$
$$\therefore \quad P = 37.4 \text{ W}$$

During transient conditions such as pulsed operation, overloads or faults, the temperature rise may be estimated by using a quantity referred to as the transient thermal impedance which incorporates the effects of thermal capacitance. This transient thermal impedance is a time-dependent function and relates the device temperature rise to the energy input in a defined time interval. For a sudden increase in dissipation at time $t = 0$ from 0 to P_{th}:

This illustrates the limitation of the analogy as impedance in electrical engineering is a steady-state term.

$$P_{th} Z_{th}(t) = \delta\theta(t) \qquad (1.4)$$

where $Z_{th}(t)$ is the thermal impedance at time t
and $\delta\theta(t)$ is the temperature rise at time t.

Curves of transient thermal impedance such as that shown in Fig. 1.23 are provided for individual semiconductors.

Consider a power semiconductor providing a continuous series of power pulses as in Fig. 1.24. The average junction temperature can be found from the mean power loss and the thermal impedance at $t = \infty$ as:

The transient thermal impedance for $t = \infty$ is the thermal resistance.

$$\theta_j = \theta_a + P_{mean} Z_{ja}(\infty) = \theta_a + P_{mean} R_{ja} \qquad (1.5)$$

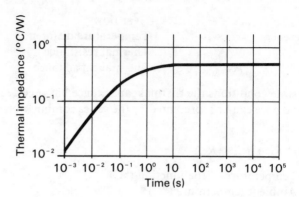

Fig. 1.23   Transient thermal impedance curve for a 100 amp thyristor.

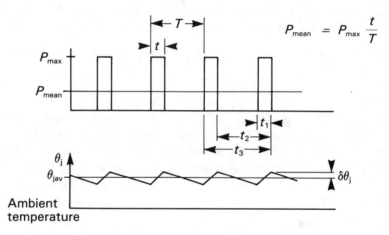

Fig. 1.24   Temperature variation with a pulsed load.

where θ_j is the junction temperature
θ_a is the ambient temperature
P_{mean} = Mean power = $P_{max} t/T$
$Z_{ja}(\infty) = R_{ja}$ = thermal impedance at $t = \infty$

The junction temperature then varies about this mean by an amount $\delta\theta_j$, a good approximation to which can be obtained by considering the last two pulses transmitted when, referring to Fig. 1.24(a):

$$\delta\theta_j = [(P_{max} - P_{mean}) Z_{th}(t_3)] - P_{max} [Z_{th}(t_2) - Z_{th}(t_1)] \qquad (1.6)$$

As the transient thermal impedance is an expression of the step response of the system it can be used directly only with waveforms that can be formed from step functions. More complex waveforms can, however, be examined by representing them as a series of step functions, with appropriate averaging, and applying the principle of superposition.

Bird, B.M. and King, K.G. (1983). *An Introduction to Power Electronics*. John Wiley, U.K.

Protection

To prevent damage to a power semiconductor device it must be protected against excessive currents and voltages and high rates of change of both current and voltage. In many cases, the selection of the protection to be employed may well owe as much to experience and practice as to formulation and analysis.

Overcurrent Protection

As the thyristor has a restricted overcurrent capacity, special fast-acting fuses are usually provided for overcurrent protection. These fuses must take account of:

(1) The need to permit the continuous passage of the steady-state current.
(2) Permitted overload conditions including transients and duty-cycle loads.
(3) Prospective fault conditions.
(4) The i^2t rating of the device. The fuse must clear the fault before the i^2t limit is reached.
(5) High peak-current levels during faults caused by current asymmetry.
(6) Fuse voltage rating.
(7) Ambient temperature conditions.

At high levels of fault current the fuse operation follows the pattern of Fig. 1.25 with operation within one cycle after time t_1. In the arcing phase, of duration t_2, the fuse is designed to present a high arc impedance in order to extinguish the arc and isolate the fault. The fuse characteristic during the melting phase is a function of the pre-arcing $\int i^2 \mathrm{d}t$ characterictic of the fuse. Conditions once the fuse is open circuit are complicated by arc voltage and current conditions; however, the total pre-arcing and arcing $\int i^2 \mathrm{d}t$ must be less than the $\int i^2 \mathrm{d}t$ rating of the device being protected.

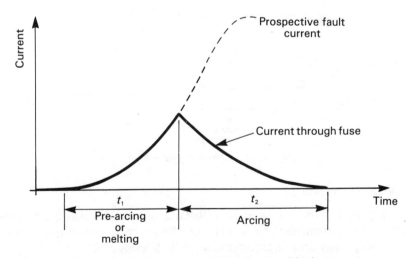

Fig. 1.25   Fuse behaviour with high levels of fault current.

At lower fault currents, fuse melting occurs more slowly and hence less explosively with the arc extinguishing at a natural current zero following melting. The melting time for the fuse will become infinite at some particular current level. This is the maximum continuous current rating of the fuse and the ratio between this current and the rated current is known as the fusing factor and would normally be of the order of 1.3 to 1.4, as is illustrated by Fig. 1.26.

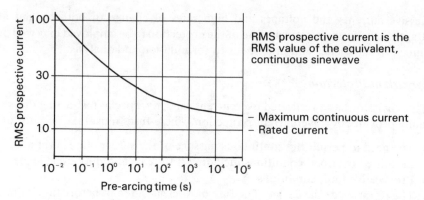

Fig. 1.26   Current-time characteristic for a 10 amp (rated) semiconductor fuse.

The overcurrent protection of transistors presents particular problems. A fault condition can cause an effective reduction in the transistor load (R_c in Fig. 1.18(c)), causing the load line of Fig. 1.19(a) to be rotated clockwise. As the supply voltage (V_s) is fixed, than for a fixed base current the transistor will come out of saturation, increasing the dissipation in the manner of Fig. 1.19(b). Though this increased dissipation may result in damage to the transistor, the rise in the collector current (I_c) may not be sufficient to blow a series fuse. To overcome this problem, the crowbar thyristor of Fig. 1.27 can be used. Here, additional circuitry is included to detect an increase in V_{CE} and fire the crowbar thyristor, causing the fuse to blow.

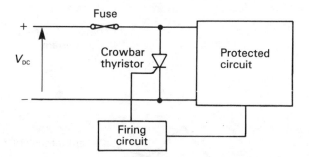

Fig. 1.27   Crowbar protection.

Overvoltage Protection

Given that the thyristor is rated to withstand the normal maximum voltages expected in the system, the problem is that of protecting against transient over-voltages, which may also be accompanied by high levels of dV/dt.

Non-linear devices having characteristics of the type shown in Fig. 1.28 can be used in parallel with the active device in company with the reactive snubber circuits of Fig. 1.13 for overvoltage protection. Three typical non-linear devices are:

Voltage-dependent resistors or varistors. These are formed from a semiconductor material such as silicon carbide (SiC) or zinc oxide (ZnO) and can provide characteristics in which the current through the varistor varies as the thirteenth or higher power of applied voltage.

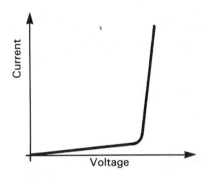

Fig. 1.28 General nonlinear surge suppressor characteristic.

Avalanche diodes. These are diodes or thyristors which can sustain large reverse currents in reverse breakdown without damage. The limitations on the use of an avalanche diode are the reverse breakdown voltage, the peak power loss and the steady-state power loss.

Selenium diode rectifiers. These are selenium-metal junction diodes constructed to have a low forward breakdown voltage and a well-defined and stable reverse breakdown voltage of around 72 V.

Applications of Power Semiconductors

The availability of power electronics devices over a wide range of currents and voltages and with a variety of switching performances has resulted in a steadily increasing number of applications which include:

DC power transmission
DC motor drives
AC motor drives
Voltage regulators
Switched-mode power supplies
Uninterruptable power supplies
Heating controls
Lighting controls

Tables 1.1 and 1.2, together with Fig. 1.29 and 1.30 summarize the applications of various power electronic devices. Each of these applications has associated with it a control option or options, the control being exercised through the variation of the switching sequences of the power electronic devices making up the circuit. In many cases, the application of microprocessor and microelectronics technologies has resulted in an expansion of the control function, as for example in the control of the DC servo motors used on robots or custom integrated circuits used for AC inverter drives.

Figures 1.30 and 1.31 are based on commercially available devices and the term 'practical amperes' represents current levels generally available commercially.

The range of control parameters used includes reference conditions such as voltage, speed, torque, position, extinction angle or current; the need to operate in conjunction with other control systems; the duration, position and frequency of the firing pulse and operation under fault conditions. Figure 1.31 sets out in diagrammatic form the basis of such a control system.

Foster, A. Mullard Ltd (1984). Trends in power semiconductors. IEE Conference Publication 234, *Power Electronics and Variable Speed Drives*.

Table 1.1   Summary of Power Electronic Technology

Aspect	Electronic power	Electrical power
Power	Low	High
Maximum frequency	High and increasing	Low and increasing
Sales quantities	High	Low
Applications	Lighting (dimmers, ballasts) Power supplies Small motors (domestic applicances) Automobile (ignition, regulator) Uninterruptable power supplies Television and audio	Induction heating Power transmission Large motors (AC or DC) Traction (automobiles, trains) Uninterruptable power supplies
Products	Thyristors Triacs Bipolar transistors and Darlingtons (high frequency) GTOs (high frequency) Power MOSFETs and Smart Power	Thyristors ASCRs Bipolar transistors and Darlingtons (high V_{CE}) GTOs
Assembly technology	Plastic packages (flat packs) Hybrids (chip assembly) Soldering, wire bonding Printed circuit boards	Plastic packages (flat pack) Stud base Capsule (hockey puck) Pressure contacts Bus bars
Quality	PPM campaigns Reliability built in Published data sometimes optimistic	Burn-in Reliability built in Published data is realistic

Foster, A. Mullard Ltd, from 'Trends in Power Semiconductors'. IEE Conference Publication 234, *Power Electronics and Variable Speed Drives*, May 1984.

Table 1.2   Relative Performance of Power Electronic Devices

Performance parameter	GTO	Bipolar	Power MOS	Bipolar-MOS hybrid
Switching speed	2	3	5	3
Switching loss	1	3	5	3
On-state loss	4	5	3	5
Blocking voltage	5	4	3	3
Surge current rating	5	3	4	4
Ease of drive	3	3	5	5
Cost	5	4	2	3
Safe operating area (SOAR)	4	3	5	3
Ease of parallel operation	3	3	5	3

Table 1.2 *cont'd*

Performance parameter	GTO	Bipolar	Power MOS	Bipolar-MOS hybrid
$\theta_{j,max}$	3	4	3	4
Gain	4	3	5	4
Chip size (high voltage)	5	3	1	4
Chip size (low voltage)	2	4	5	3

5 — Excellent
4 — Very good
3 — Good
2 — Moderate
1 — Poor

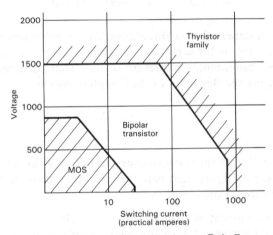

Fig. 1.29 General operating areas of power products. © A. Foster, Mullard Ltd, from 'Trends in Power Semiconductors', IEE Conf. Pub. 234, *Power Electronics and Variable Speed Drives*, May 1984.

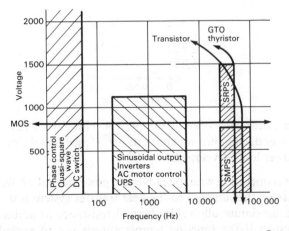

Fig. 1.30 Power electronic devices, general applications areas. © A. Foster, Mullard Ltd, from 'Trends in Power Semiconductors', IEE Conf. Pub. 234, *Power Electronics and Variable Speed Drives*, May 1984.

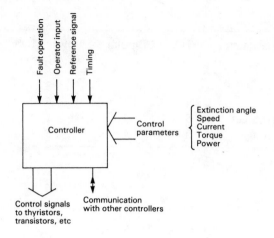

Fig. 1.31 Control system layout.

A current development is the incorporation of intelligence alongside the switching circuit, either on the same chip or as part of a hybrid circuit. Such *smart power* components can monitor and report on their status and regulate their own operation, increasing the flexibility of the complete system.

Problems

1.1 An approximation to the forward characteristic of a thyristor is as shown in the accompanying figure. Estimate the mean power loss in the thyristor for the following conditions.

(a) A constant current of 52 A for one-half cycle.
(b) A constant current of 22 A for one-third of a cycle.
(c) A constant current of 44 A for two-thirds of a cycle.

What will be the RMS current rating for each of the above load conditions?

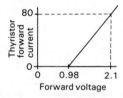

1.2 For the transistor of Worked Example 1.4, plot curves showing the instantaneous power during turn-on and turn-off. Hence find the maximum instantaneous power level developed.

1.3 A thyristor is operating with a steady-state power loss of 32 W. If the thermal resistance from the junction to the heat transfer system is 0.81°C/W, what will be the maximum allowable thermal resistance to ambient of the heat transfer system if the junction temperature is not to exceed 130°C at an ambient temperature of 42°C?

What will be the thyristor base temperature under these conditions?

1.4 A thyristor with the transient thermal impedance characteristic of Fig. 1.23 is supplying a pulsed load such as that shown in Fig. 1.24, with $P_{max} = 48$ W; $t = 20$ ms; $T = 100$ ms.

Estimate the maximum junction temperature of the thyristor if the ambient temperature is 24°C.

1.5 Two diodes having approximate characteristics in the forward direction:

Diode 1 $v = 0.88 + 2.44 \times 10^{-4}, i$
Diode 2 $v = 0.96 + 2.32 \times 10^{-4}, i$

are connected in parallel. Find the current in each diode if the total current is (a) 400, (b) 800, (c) 1200, (d) 1600 and (e) 2000 A.

What single value of resistance connected in series with each diode will bring the diode currents to within 8% of equal current sharing with a total current of 1200 A? How will this affect the current sharing at total currents of 400 and 2000 A?

1.6 A string of three thyristors connected in series as in Fig. 1.12(b) is designed to withstand an off-state voltage of 7.2 kV. If the compensating circuit components have values of $R_1 = 30$ Ω, $R_2 = 24\ 000$ Ω and $C = 0.088$ μF, estimate the voltage across each thyristor in the off state and the discharge current of each capacitor on turn-on. The leakages currents for the thyristors are $T_1 = 18$ mA, $T_2 = 24$ mA and $T_3 = 16$ mA.

2 Converters

Objectives
- [ ] To understand what is meant by operation of a converter in the rectifying and inverting modes.
- [ ] To examine the operation of naturally commutated converters.
- [ ] To consider the operation of uncontrolled, fully-controlled and half-controlled converters.
- [ ] To develop the general equations describing converter behaviour.
- [ ] To understand the effect of firing delay and extinction angles on converter performance.
- [ ] To examine the effect of source inductance on commutation and to define overlap.
- [ ] To consider the function and operation of the freewheeling diode.
- [ ] To define power factor in relation to a converter circuit.

Rectification

Rectification is the process of converting a bi-directional (alternating) current or voltage into a uni-directional (direct) current or voltage. This conversion can be achieved by a variety of circuits based on and using any of the switching devices discussed in Chapter 1, with the use of diodes probably the most familiar. By using thyristors, power transistors, power MOS, etc., additional control over the magnitude of the direct voltage can be achieved by varying the point-on-wave at which the device is placed into the conducting state. In this chapter, the operation of rectifiers and converters ranging from a simple half-wave rectifier using a single diode to complex multi-phase, full-wave bridge circuits employing several thyristors will be considered.

The point-on-wave at which a thyristor is fired is defined by the firing angle α.

The rectifier circuits can be separated broadly into three classes; uncontrolled, fully-controlled and half-controlled. An uncontrolled rectifier uses only diodes and the DC output voltage is fixed in amplitude by the amplitude of the AC supply. The fully-controlled rectifier uses thyristors as the rectifying elements and the DC output voltage is a function of the amplitude of the AC supply voltage and the point-on-wave at which the thyristors are fired. The half-controlled rectifier contains a mixture of diodes and thyristors, allowing a more limited control of the DC output voltage level than the fully-controlled rectifier. The half-controlled rectifier is cheaper than a fully-controlled rectifier of the same rating but has operational limitations.

A six-pulse converter operating from a 50 Hz supply produces a 300 Hz (6 × 50) ripple in the output DC voltage waveform.

Rectifiers are often described by their pulse number. This is the number of discrete switching operations involving load transfer (commutation) between individual diodes, thyristors, etc, during one cycle of the AC supply waveform. The pulse number is therefore directly related to the repetition period of the DC voltage waveform and is sometimes expressed in terms of the ripple frequency of this waveform.

Inversion

Uncontrolled and half-controlled rectifiers will permit power to flow only from the AC system to the DC load and are therefore referred to as unidirectional converters. However, with a fully-controlled rectifier it is possible, by control of the point-on-wave at which switching takes place, to allow power to be transferred from the DC side of the rectifier back into the AC system. When this occurs, operation is said to be in the inverting mode. The fully-controlled converter may therefore be referred to as a bi-directional converter.

Commutating Diode

It was shown in Chapter 1 that if a thyristor or diode is used to supply an inductive load, then the load voltage will reverse during the conduction interval. This condition is shown in Fig. 2.1(a). The commutating or freewheeling diode of Fig. 2.1(b) is used, particularly with uncontrolled or half-controlled converters, to prevent this voltage reversal. Also, by transferring current from the main converter, the commutating diode allows the main thyristors and diodes to resume their blocking state. The current through the commutating diode is maintained by the energy stored in the magnetic field of the load inductance.

The load voltage will in fact reverse by an amount equal to the forward voltage drop of the commutating diode.

Naturally Commutated Thyristor Converters

Figure 2.2(a) shows a full-wave rectifier using diodes, while Fig. 2.2(b) has the same circuit but with the diodes replaced by thyristors. The point-on-wave at which the thyristors are fired is defined by the firing angle α and is measured from the point at which an ideal diode replacing the thyristor would begin to conduct. This definition of firing angle is applied to all the thyristor converters considered. The response of the equivalent diode circuits, thyristors replaced by diodes, can therefore be obtained by putting $\alpha = 0°$.

Also referred to as the bi-phase, half-wave rectifier.

Also referred to as the firing delay or delay angle.

The diode-only circuits form the uncontrolled converters.

For the circuit of Fig. 2.2(b), an inductive load has been assumed such that load current is continuous. At the instant of firing thyristor T_2, with thyristor T_1 conducting, the positive voltage v_2 appears across the load. This results in a current transfer between thyristors T_1 and T_2, at the end of which T_2 has assumed the load current and T_1 has been commutated off. The mean load voltage is obtained by averaging the rectifier output voltage over the conduction interval.

This is typical of loads such as large motors.

$$V_{mean} = \frac{1}{\pi} \int_{\alpha}^{\alpha + \pi} V_m \sin \omega t \, d(\omega t) = (2V_m \cos \alpha)/\pi \qquad (2.1)$$

Figure 2.3 shows the circuits and waveforms for both the single-phase fully-controlled and half-controlled bridges. The effect of the commutating diode in preventing the reversal of the load voltage can be seen from the accompanying output voltage waveforms. The conduction period of the fully-controlled bridge is π and that of the half-controlled bridge is $\pi - \alpha$ as a result of the action of the commutating diode. The load voltages, ignoring thyristor and diode voltage drops, are:

For a practical (non-ideal) thyristor the mean voltage will be reduced by the thyristor forward voltage drop.

$$V'_{mean} = V_{mean} - V_{thyristor}$$

Compare the waveforms of Fig. 2.3(a) with those of Fig. 2.2(b).

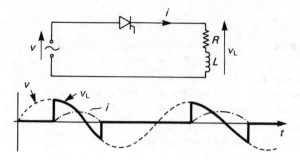

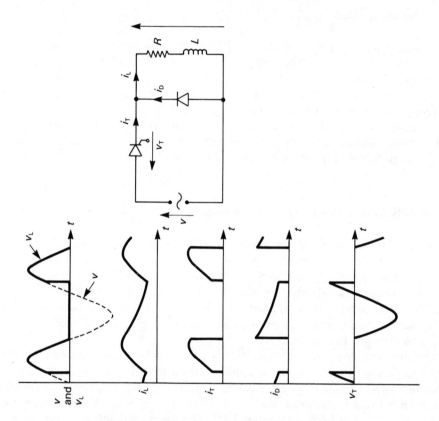

Fig. 2.1a Thyristor with inductive load.

Fig. 2.1b Effect of commutating diode.

Fully-controlled bridge

V_m is the peak amplitude of the single-phase supply voltage.

$$V_{\text{mean}} = \frac{1}{\pi} \int_{\alpha}^{\alpha + \pi} V_m \sin(\omega t)\, d(\omega t) = (2V_m \cos \alpha)/\pi \tag{2.2}$$

Half-controlled bridge

$$V_{\text{mean}} = \frac{1}{\pi} \int_{\alpha}^{\pi} V_m \sin(\omega t)\, d(\omega t) = V_m(1 + \cos \alpha)/\pi \tag{2.3}$$

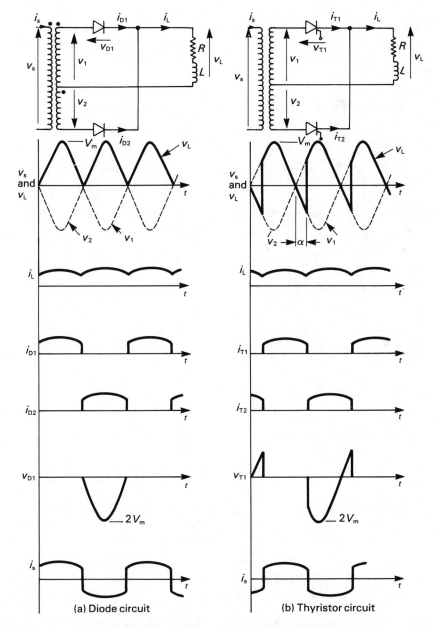

Fig. 2.2   Single phase full wave rectifier circuits.

A highly inductive load, such that the load current can be assumed constant, is to be supplied from a 240 V, 50 Hz, single-phase supply by a fully-controlled and a half-controlled bridge. Compare the mean load voltage provided by each bridge at firing angles of 30° and 90°. Ignore device voltage drops.

Worked Example 2.1

For the fully-controlled bridge

$$V_{\text{mean},30°} = \frac{2 \times 240 \times \sqrt{2}}{\pi} \cos 30° = 187.1 \text{ V}$$

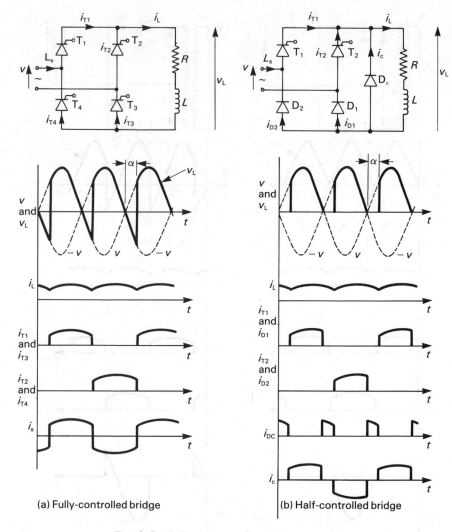

Fig. 2.3 Full wave rectifier bridge circuits.

$$V_{\text{mean},90°} = \frac{2 \times 240 \times \sqrt{2}}{\pi} \cos 90° = 0 \text{ V}$$

From Fig. 2.9(b) it can be seen that for the fully-controlled bridge with a firing angle of 90°, the positive and negative components of the load voltage are equal, giving a mean voltage of zero.

For the half-controlled bridge

$$V_{\text{mean},30°} = \frac{240 \times \sqrt{2}}{\pi} (1 + \cos 30°) = 201.6 \text{ V}$$

$$V_{\text{mean},90°} = \frac{240 \times \sqrt{2}}{\pi} (1 + \cos 90°) = 108 \text{ V}$$

The difference in the mean voltages of the fully and half-controlled bridges is a

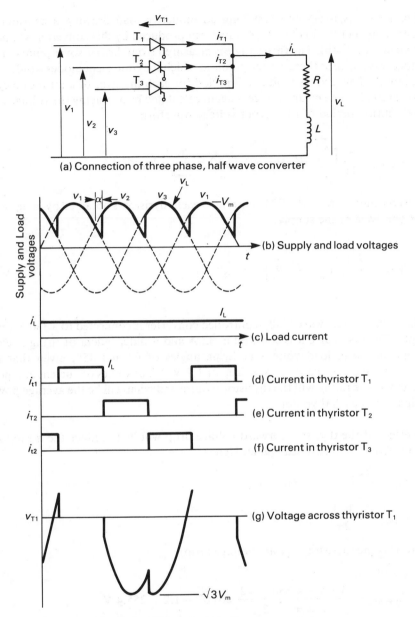

(a) Connection of three phase, half wave converter

(b) Supply and load voltages

(c) Load current

(d) Current in thyristor T₁

(e) Current in thyristor T₂

(f) Current in thyristor T₃

(g) Voltage across thyristor T₁

Fig. 2.4   Three phase half wave converter.

result of the action of the commutating diode in preventing the reversal of load voltage.

Single-phase converters are limited to powers of a few kilowatts. Where higher power levels are required, converters based on polyphase supplies are used. The three-phase, half-wave circuit of Fig. 2.4(a) forms the basis of many of these circuits.

See appendix for details of three-phase systems.

For ideal thyristors and assuming an inductive load drawing a continuous, constant current the load voltage waveform produced by this converter will be as shown in Fig. 2.4(b). The firing angle is measured from the crossover points of the voltage waveform as these are the points at which the equivalent diodes would start to conduct. This gives a conduction period for each thyristor of a third of a cycle (120° or $2\pi/3$). The mean voltage is again calculated by averaging the voltage over the repetition period of the output voltage waveform.

V_m is the amplitude of the phase voltage of the three-phase supply.

$$V_{mean} = \frac{3}{2\pi} \int_{\frac{\pi}{6}+\alpha}^{\frac{5\pi}{6}+\alpha} V_m \sin(\omega t)\, d(\omega t) = \frac{3\sqrt{3}}{2\pi} V_m \cos\alpha \qquad (2.4)$$

For a constant current, the RMS current in each thyristor is obtained by integrating over one cycle of the supply.

$$I_{RMS} = \left[\frac{1}{2\pi} \int_{\alpha}^{\alpha+\frac{2\pi}{3}} I_L^2\, d\theta \right]^{\frac{1}{2}} = \frac{I_L}{3} \qquad (2.5)$$

Worked Example 2.2

A three-phase, half-wave, fully-controlled converter is connected to a 380 V (line) supply. The load current is constant at 32 A and is independent of firing angle.

Find the mean load voltage at firing angles of 0° and 45°, given that the thyristors have a forward voltage drop of 1.2 V. What values of current and peak reverse voltage rating will the thyristor require and what will be the average power dissipation in each thyristor?

The effect of the thyristor forward voltage drop will be to reduce the mean load voltage from the theoretical value. Hence

$$V_m = \frac{380 \times \sqrt{2}}{\sqrt{3}} = 310.3 \text{ V}$$

$$V_{mean} = \frac{3\sqrt{3}}{2\pi} V_m \cos\alpha - V_t$$

where V_t is the thyristor forward voltage drop.

$\alpha = 0°$

$$V_{mean,0°} = \frac{3 \times \sqrt{3} \times 380 \times \sqrt{2}}{2 \times \pi \times \sqrt{3}} \cos 0° - 1.2 = 255.4 \text{ V}$$

$\alpha = 45°$

$$V_{mean,45°} = \frac{3 \times \sqrt{3} \times 380 \times \sqrt{2}}{2 \times \pi \times \sqrt{3}} \cos 45° - 1.2 = 180.2 \text{ V}$$

Ratings

$$I_{RMS} = 32/\sqrt{3} = 18.47 \text{ A}$$

From Fig. 2.4 the reverse voltage can be seen to be the difference between the two phase voltages, i.e. the line voltage of the three-phase supply. The peak reverse voltage (PRV) is therefore the peak value of the AC line voltage.

$$PRV = \sqrt{2}\, V_{line} = \sqrt{2} \times \sqrt{3} \times V_{phase} = \sqrt{2} \times 380 = 537.4 \text{ V}$$

The average power dissipated in the thyristor is obtained by averaging the instantaneous power dissipation over one cycle. This gives

$$\text{Average power} = \frac{1}{2\pi} \int_{\alpha}^{\alpha + \frac{2\pi}{3}} v_t i_t \, d\theta = \frac{V_t I_t}{3} = \frac{1.2 \times 32}{3}$$
$$= 12.8 \text{ W}$$

Overlap

So far no account has been taken of the effect of source impedance on converter behaviour. Consider the three-phase, half-wave bridge at the instant of firing thyristor T_2. With a constant load current the effect of firing T_2 is to set up a circulating current between thyristors T_1 and T_2 as shown in Fig. 2.5. This circulating current will increase from zero at the instant of firing T_2 until it equals the load current I_L, at which point the current in T_1 becomes zero and this thyristor is turned off and commutation is completed. The interval during which both thyristors are conducting is referred to as the overlap period and is defined by the overlap angle γ. This angle may be calculated by reference to Fig. 2.5 when, ignoring thyristor voltage drops:

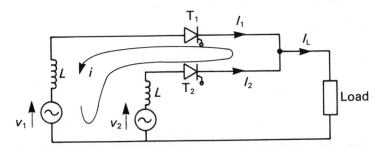

Fig. 2.5   Commutation between thyristor T_1 and T_2 including source inductance.

$$v_2 - v_1 = 2L \, di/dt \tag{2.6}$$

Putting $t = 0$ at the instant of firing T_2, then

$$v_2 - v_1 = v_{line} = \sqrt{3} \, V_m \sin(\omega t + \alpha) \tag{2.7}$$

Combining Equations 2.6 and 2.7

$$di = \frac{\sqrt{3} \, V_m}{2L} \sin(\omega t + \alpha) \, dt$$

Integrating this equation from $t = 0$ to t

$$i = \frac{\sqrt{3} \, V_m}{2\omega L} \{\cos \alpha - \cos(\omega t + \alpha)\} \tag{2.8}$$

Commutation is complete when $i = I_L$, i.e. when $\omega t = \gamma$. Hence

$$I_L = \frac{\sqrt{3} \, V_m}{2\omega L} [\cos \alpha - \cos(\gamma + \alpha)] \tag{2.9}$$

Thyristor currents during commutation.
Load current $= I_L = |i_1 - i_2|$

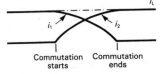

35

Since both thyristors are
conducting together. Assumes
identical source inductance
values.

During commutation the load voltage will be the mean of v_1 and v_2, resulting in a change in the mean voltage of the load to

$$V_{\text{mean}} = \frac{3}{2\pi} \left\{ \int_{\alpha + \gamma + \frac{\pi}{6}}^{\alpha + \frac{5\pi}{6}} V_m \sin(\omega t)\, d(\omega t) \right.$$

$$\left. + \frac{1}{2} \int_{\alpha + \frac{\pi}{6}}^{\alpha + \gamma + \frac{\pi}{6}} V_m \left[\sin\left(\omega t + \frac{2\pi}{3}\right) + \sin \omega t \right] d(\omega t) \right\}$$

$$= \frac{3\sqrt{3}\, V_m}{4\pi} \{\cos\alpha + \cos(\alpha + \gamma)\} \tag{2.10}$$

ΔV_d is the change in rectifier
output voltage due to overlap.

Now let $V_{\text{mean}} = V_0 - \Delta V_d$ and from Equation 2.4

$$V_0 = \frac{3\sqrt{3}}{2\pi} V_m \cos\alpha$$

Hence

$$\Delta V_d = \frac{3\sqrt{3}}{4\pi} V_m \{\cos\alpha - \cos(\alpha + \gamma)\} \tag{2.11}$$

Combining Equations 2.9 and 2.11

$$\Delta V_d = \frac{3\omega L}{2\pi} I_L \tag{2.12}$$

From Equations 2.10 and 2.12

$$V_{\text{mean}} = \frac{3\sqrt{3}}{2\pi} V_m \cos\alpha - \frac{3\omega L}{2\pi} I_L = V_0 - R_r I_L \tag{2.13}$$

The ΔV_d term can therefore be considered in terms of an effective DC resistance component R_r and the load current I_L. The rectifier can then be represented by the equivalent circuit of Fig. 2.6. It is important to note that the resistance term R_r in this circuit represents a voltage drop *only*, and *not* a power loss. Device forward voltage drops and lead resistances could also be included in this equivalent circuit when they would represent *both* a voltage drop *and* a power loss.

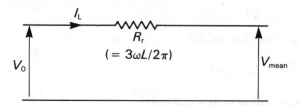

Fig. 2.6   Basic circuit for three phase half wave converter in rectifying mode.

Figure 2.7 shows the effect of overlap on the output voltage, phase currents and source voltage of a three-phase, half-wave rectifier.

Worked Example 2.3

A single-phase, full-wave converter as shown in the figure is supplied from a 120 V,

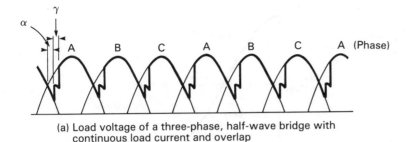

(a) Load voltage of a three-phase, half-wave bridge with
continuous load current and overlap

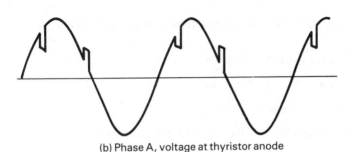

(b) Phase A, voltage at thyristor anode

Fig. 2.7   Operation of a three phase half wave bridge with overlap.

50 Hz supply with a source inductance of 0.333 mH. Assuming the load current is
continuous at 4 A, find the overlap angles for (i) transfer of current from a
conducting thyristor to the commutating diode and (ii) from the commutating
diode to a thyristor when the firing angle is 15°.

Single-phase, full-wave
converter with commutating
diode.

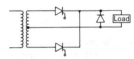

Commutation from thyristor to diode begins at time $t = 0$, the instant when the
load voltage starts to reverse (ignoring device voltage drops). Hence at the onset of
commutation and referring to the figure,

Commutation from thyristor to
diode.

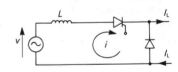

$$v = -V_m \sin \omega t = -L \, di/dt$$

From this equation

$$di = V_m \sin (\omega t) \, dt/L$$

Integrating

$$i = \frac{V_m}{L} \int_0^t \sin \omega t \, (dt)$$

$$= \frac{V_m}{\omega L} (1 - \cos \omega t)$$

Commutation is complete when $i = I_L$, at which point $\omega t = \gamma_1$.
   Thus

$$I_L = \frac{V_m}{\omega L} (1 - \cos \gamma_1)$$

Solving using the values given, $\gamma_1 = 4.02°$
Commutation from the diode to the thyristor begins at the instant of firing the
thyristor. Putting $t = 0$ at the instant of firing then, referring to the figure:

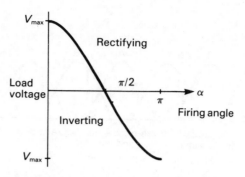

Fig. 2.8   Variation of mean load voltage with firing angle.

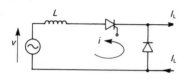

$$v = V_m \sin (\omega t + \alpha) = L \, di/dt$$

After integrating as before, this gives

$$i = V_m [\cos \alpha - \cos (\omega t - \alpha)]/\omega L$$

Commutation is complete when $i = I_L$ and $\omega t = \gamma_2$, when

$$I_L = V_m[\cos \alpha - \cos (\gamma_2 + \alpha)]/\omega L$$

Substituting values gives, $\gamma_2 = 0.536°$

Inversion

Figure 2.8 shows the curve of mean load voltage against firing angle for a three-phase, half-wave converter in the absence of overlap. For firing angles greater than 90° this mean voltage becomes negative and, since the direction of current through the thyristors cannot reverse the direction of power flow, is now from the DC side of the converter back into the AC supply. The converter is now operating in the inverting mode. Figure 2.9 shows the load voltage waveforms for the three-phase, half-wave converter at various firing angles.

Commutation between any pair of thyristors will occur only if the instantaneous anode voltage of the thyristor being turned on is greater than that of the conducting thyristor throughout the whole of the overlap period. If this is not the case and the two commutating voltages become first equal and then reverse before the current transfer is complete, then the current will revert to the initially conducting thyristor. This situation for a converter operating in the inverting mode is illustrated by Fig. 2.10.

When the converter is operating in the inverting mode, the point-on-wave at which a thyristor is fired is defined more usually by reference to the firing advance angle β rather than the firing delay angle α. The relationship between α and β is

$$\beta = 180° - \alpha \qquad (2.14)$$

and applies to converters of any pulse number.

The effect of overlap and the need to maintain a higher instantaneous voltage on the incoming thyristor modifies the conditions near the limit ($\alpha = 180°$). For this reason an extinction angle δ is specified such that

$$\delta = \beta - \gamma \qquad (2.15)$$

38

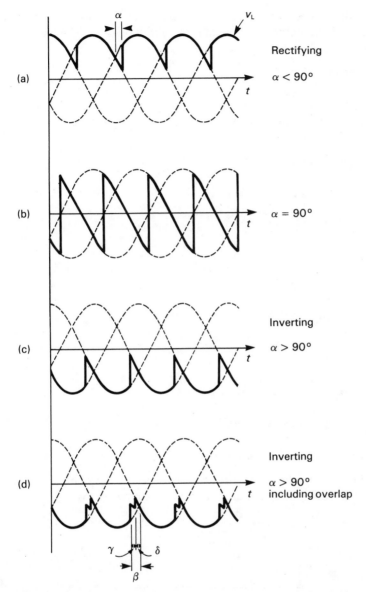

Fig. 2.9 Three phase half wave converter showing effect of firing angle variation.

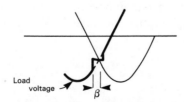

Fig. 2.10 Commutation failure in inverting mode due to voltage reversal before commutation is complete.

See Figs. 2.9 and 2.10.

with δ usually limited to a minimum value of about 5° to ensure commutation and a reversion to the full blocking state before voltage reversal. The DC mean voltage, assuming constant current, is:

Ignoring overlap

$$V_{\text{mean}} = \frac{3}{2\pi} \int_{\frac{\pi}{6}-\beta}^{\frac{5\pi}{6}-\beta} V_{\text{m}} \sin \omega t \, d(\omega t) = \frac{3\sqrt{3}}{2\pi} V_{\text{m}} \cos \omega t = V_0 \tag{2.16}$$

Including overlap

$$V_{\text{mean}} = \frac{3}{2\pi} \left\{ \int_{\frac{\pi}{6}+\gamma-\beta}^{\frac{5\pi}{6}-\beta} V_{\text{m}} \sin \omega t \, d(\omega t) \right.$$

$$\left. + \frac{1}{2} \int_{\frac{\pi}{6}-\beta}^{\frac{\pi}{6}+\gamma-\beta} V_{\text{m}} \left[\sin \left(\omega t + \frac{2\pi}{3} \right) + \sin \omega t \right] d(\omega t) \right\}$$

$$= \frac{3\sqrt{3}}{4\pi} V_{\text{m}} [\cos \beta + \cos (\beta - \gamma)] \tag{2.17}$$

Now let

$$V_{\text{mean}} = V_0 + \Delta V_{\text{d}} \tag{2.18}$$

Compare with equivalent calculation using Equations 2.9 to 2.11 for rectifier.

Compare with Equation 2.13.

Combining Equations 2.9, 2.16, 2.17 and 2.18

$$V_{\text{mean}} = \frac{3\sqrt{3}}{2\pi} V_{\text{m}} \cos \beta + \frac{3\omega L}{2\pi} I_{\text{L}} = V_0 + R_{\text{i}} I_{\text{L}} \tag{2.19}$$

where $\Delta V_{\text{d}} = R_{\text{i}} I_{\text{L}}$ and $R_{\text{i}} = 3\omega L / 2\pi$

Equation 2.19 can be represented by the inverter equivalent circuit of Fig. 2.11 with R_{i} representing a voltage drop *only* and *not* a power loss.

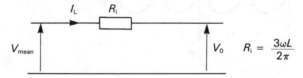

Fig. 2.11   Equivalent circuit for three phase half wave converter in inverting mode.

Worked Example 2.4

A three-phase, half-wave converter is operating in the inverting mode connected to a 415 V (line) supply. If the extinction angle is 18° and the overlap 3.8° find the mean voltage at the load.

Using Equation 2.17

$$V_{\text{mean}} = \frac{3\sqrt{3}}{4\pi} \times \frac{415\sqrt{2}}{\sqrt{3}} \times (\cos 18° + \cos 14.2°) = 269.1 \text{ V}$$

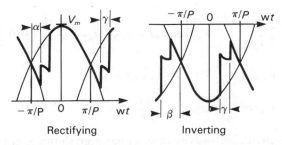

Fig. 2.12 Output voltage waveforms for a p-pulse converter.

Converter equations

The converter equations developed so far have been for the three-pulse, three-phase, half-wave converter. Similar analyses can be used to develop the equations for a general p-pulse, fully-controlled converter. Referring to Fig. 2.12:

Rectifying
Ignoring overlap:

$$V_0 = \frac{p}{2\pi} \int_{\alpha - \frac{\pi}{p}}^{\alpha + \frac{\pi}{p}} V_m \cos(\omega t)\, d(\omega t) = \frac{p}{\pi} V_m \sin(\pi/p) \cos\alpha \qquad (2.20)$$

Including overlap:

$$\begin{aligned}
V_{\text{mean}} &= \frac{p}{2\pi} \left\{ \int_{\alpha + \gamma - \frac{\pi}{p}}^{\alpha + \frac{\pi}{p}} V_m \cos(\omega t)\, d(\omega t) \right. \\
&\quad \left. + \frac{1}{2} \int_{\alpha - \frac{\pi}{p}}^{\alpha + \gamma - \frac{\pi}{p}} V_m \left[\cos(\omega t) + \cos\left(\omega t + \frac{2\pi}{3}\right) \right] d(\omega t) \right\} \\
&= \frac{p}{2\pi} V_m \sin\left(\frac{\pi}{p}\right) [\cos\alpha + \cos(\alpha + \gamma)] \\
&= \frac{p}{\pi} V_m \sin\left(\frac{\pi}{p}\right) \cos\alpha - \frac{p\omega L}{2p} I_L \qquad (2.21)
\end{aligned}$$

Inverting
Ignoring overlap:

$$V_0 = \frac{p}{2\pi} \int_{-\beta - \frac{\pi}{p}}^{-\beta + \frac{\pi}{p}} V_m \cos(\omega t)\, d(\omega t) = \frac{p}{\pi} V_m \sin(\pi/p) \cos\beta \qquad (2.22)$$

Including overlap:

$$V_{\text{mean}} = \frac{p}{2\pi} \left\{ \int_{-\beta - \frac{\pi}{p} + \gamma}^{-\beta + \frac{\pi}{p}} V_m \cos(\omega t)\, d(\omega t) \right.$$

$$+ \frac{1}{2} \int_{-\beta-\frac{\pi}{p}}^{-\beta-\frac{\pi}{p}+\gamma} V_m \left[\cos \omega t + \cos \left(\omega t + \frac{2\pi}{3} \right) \right] d(\omega t) \Bigg\}$$

$$= \frac{p}{2\pi} V_m \sin \left(\frac{\pi}{p} \right) [\cos \beta + \cos (\beta + \gamma)]$$

$$= \frac{p}{\pi} V_m \sin \left(\frac{\pi}{p} \right) \cos \beta + \frac{p\omega L}{2\pi} I_L \tag{2.23}$$

So far, the three-phase, half-wave converter has been shown as connected directly to the three-phase supply. In practice, the converter will often be supplied via a transformer. If a simple star–star transformer, such as is shown in Fig. 2.13, were used then a unidirectional current will flow in each phase and may result in DC magnetization of the transformer core. In order to prevent this occuring the inter-connected star winding of Fig. 2.14 is used, in which a bi-directional current flows in each of the primary windings.

See appendix for details of three-phase systems.

Also referred to as a star-zigzag transformer.

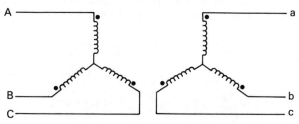

Fig. 2.13   Star-star transformer.

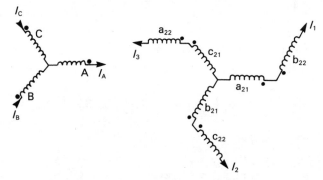

Windings a_{21} and a_{22} couple with winding A etc

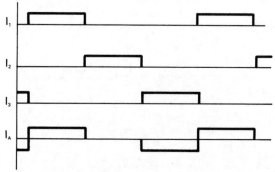

Fig. 2.14   Interconnected star winding.

42

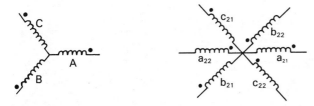

Fig. 2.15 Transformers configuration giving an effective 6-phase output.

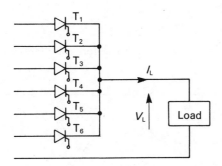

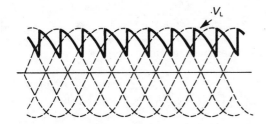

Fig. 2.16 Six-phase half wave, fully converted converter.

If the transformer connection of Fig. 2.15 is used an effective six-phase supply can be obtained which can be used with the six-phase, half-wave converter of Fig. 2.16. In practice, this simple transformer connection, in which current flows in each leg of the primary winding for only one third of a cycle, is not normally used, as it introduces high levels of harmonic current into the primary system. To reduce the levels of primary harmonic current the star-fork connection of Fig. 2.17 is used in which current flows in each phase of the primary winding for two-thirds of a cycle.

Such unconventional transformer windings are expensive and the arrangement of Fig. 2.18 may be used instead. Here, the star points of the two sets of secondary windings have been connected by an interphase reactor or transformer. Each group of thyristors (T_1, T_3, T_5 and T_2, T_4, T_6) then operates as a conventional three-phase, half-wave bridge, with each thyristor conducting for 120°. Under these conditions the load voltage is the mean of the voltages of the individual three-phase groups as shown in Fig. 2.18(b). The potential difference across the interphase reactor is the difference between the voltages of the individual three-phase groups.

The action of the interphase reactor depends on the presence of a magnetizing current which flows between the star points, causing a slight imbalance between the currents in each half of the reactor. The return magnetizing current passes via the

The DOT convention is used with mutually coupled coils to relate the sense of the induced voltage to the source current. For current direction as shown the voltage in the coupled coil has the polarity indicated.

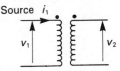

In Fig. 2.16 and subsequently, overlap is ignored for clarity and simplicity. It is present in any real circuit.

Third-harmonic current in the circuit of Fig. 2.15 has an amplitude of $4I_L/3\pi$. Third-harmonic current in the circuit of Fig. 2.17 is zero. Assumes no overlap and a constant load current.

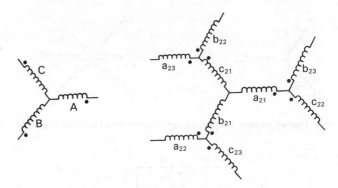

Fig. 2.17 Star-fork transformer connection.

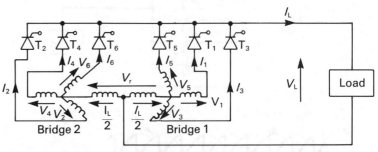

(a) Converter with interphase reactor

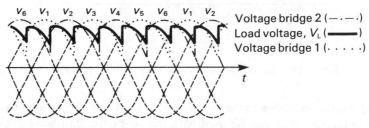

(b) Output of bridge circuits and load voltage

Voltage bridge 2 (— · — ·)
Load voltage, V_L (——)
Voltage bridge 1 (· · · · ·)

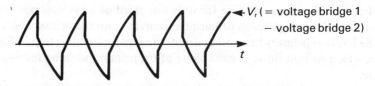

V_r (= voltage bridge 1
— voltage bridge 2)

(c) Reactor Voltage V_r

Fig. 2.18 Converter with interphase reactor.

conducting thyristor in each bridge, in one case as a reverse current. To allow this magnetizing current to flow the load current must be greater than the magnetizing current. Therefore a converter of this type is often operated into a permanently connected load which draws a current in excess of the magnetizing current to ensure correct operation of the converter for all added loads.

Figure 2.19 shows two three-phase, half-wave bridge circuits connected to operate off the positive and negative half cycles of the supply waveform respectively. This is the familiar three-phase, 6-pulse bridge circuit, more

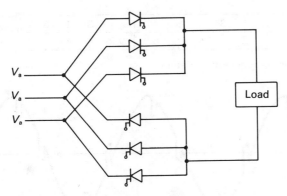

Fig. 2.19   Three phase full wave converter formed by connection of two three phase half wave converters.

commonly drawn as in Fig. 2.20. Each thyristor conducts for 120°, with a commutation taking place every 60°.

Since in normal operation two thyristors are conducting together an appropriate pair of thyristors must be gated together to initiate operation of the converter. In practice this means that one thyristor is always supplied with two firing signals 60°

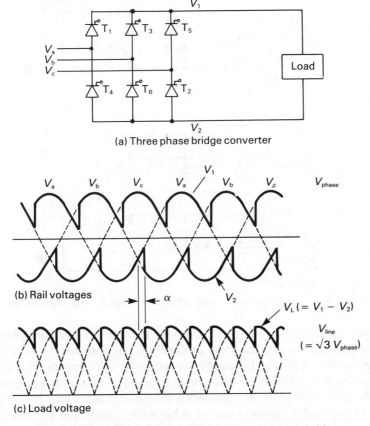

(a) Three phase bridge converter

(b) Rail voltages

(c) Load voltage

Fig. 2.20   Operation of the three phase converter bridge.

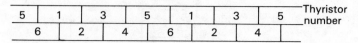

(d) Firing sequence of thyristors

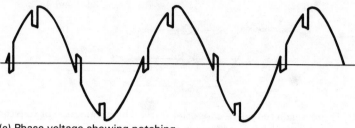

(e) Phase voltage showing notching
caused by overlap

Fig. 2.20   cont'd

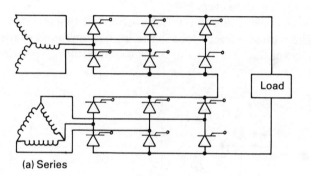

(a) Series

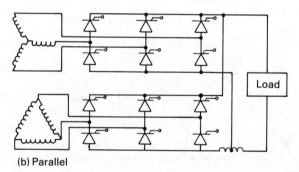

(b) Parallel

Fig. 2.21   12-pulse bridge configurations using 2 × 6-phase bridges.

apart, the second signal having no effect on this thyristor once bridge operation has been initiated and the thyristors are conducting. For applications such as power DC transmission, higher pulse number circuits may well be required. Figure 2.21 shows two ways in which two 6-pulse bridges can be combined using transformers with a 30° phase shift between secondary windings to produce an effective 12-pulse bridge. Higher pulse numbers can be achieved by combining the basic 6-pulse converter circuit with varying transformer phase shifts.

A DC link consists of two 6-pulse, fully-controlled bridge converters of the type shown in Fig. 2.20(a) connected by a transmission line of 0.2 Ω resistance and used to connect a three-phase, 415 V (line), 50 Hz system to a three-phase, 380 V (line), 60 Hz system. The source inductance of the 50 Hz system is 1 mH/phase and that of the 60 Hz system 1.25 mH/phase.

Worked Example 2.5

If the DC, link is carrying a constant DC current of 50 A and delivering 15 kW into the 60 Hz system, find the firing advance angle of the inverter and the firing angle of the rectifier.

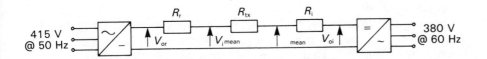

The basic rectifier and inverter equivalent circuits of Fig. 2.6 and 2.11 can be combined with the DC link resistance to give the system equivalent circuit shown. The values of R_r and R_i can then be calculated from the given data.

Compare with Fig. 2.6.

Note frequencies used in calculating R_i and R_r.

$$R_r = \frac{6 \times 100 \times \pi \times 10^{-3}}{2\pi} = 0.3 \ \Omega$$

$$R_i = \frac{6 \times 120 \times \pi \times 1.25 \times 10^{-3}}{2\pi} = 0.45 \ \Omega$$

For the inverter the mean voltage can be found from the power flow and DC current.

$$V_{mean,i} = \frac{1500}{50} = 300 \ V$$

The mean voltage in the absence of overlap can then be found

$$V_{0,i} = V_{mean,i} - R_i I_L = 300 - (50 \times 0.45) = 277.5 \ V$$

Using Equation 2.2 with $p = 6$ and V_m = Peak value of the line voltage:

$$\cos \beta = \frac{V_{0,i}}{V_{m,i}} \times \frac{\pi}{p \sin(\pi/p)} = \frac{277.5 \times \pi}{380 \times \sqrt{2} \times 6 \times \sin 30°} = 0.5408$$

Hence

$$\beta = 48.53°$$

The rectifier mean voltage, including overlap, can now be found

$$V_{mean,r} = V_{mean,i} + R_t I_L = 300 + (50 \times 0.2) = 310 \ V$$

The mean voltage, ignoring overlap can then be obtained using the load current and R_r.

$$V_{0,r} = V_{mean,r} + I_L R_r = 310 + (50 \times 0.3) = 325 \ V$$

Using Equation 2.20 with $p = 6$

$$\cos \alpha = \frac{V_{0,r}}{V_{m,r}} \times \frac{\pi}{p \sin(\pi/p)} = \frac{325\pi}{415 \times \sqrt{2} \times 6 \times \sin 30°} = 0.5799$$

Hence

$$\alpha = 54.56°$$

See Fig. 2.3(b).

The majority of the converters considered so far have been fully controlled or, by putting $\alpha = 0°$, the equivalent uncontrolled converter. Figures 2.3(b) and 2.22 show the circuits and waveforms for single- and three-phase, half-controlled converter bridges. In each case the thyristors commutate on when fired and are commutated off either on the firing of another thyristor or by the action of the commutating diode.

Consider the three-phase, half-controlled bridge converter. When the firing angle is $\leqslant 60°$, the commutating diode plays no part and each thyristor and diode conducts for a full 120°. Under these conditions the mean load voltage is:

V_m is the peak amplitude of the AC line voltage.

$$V_{mean} = \frac{3}{2\pi}\left[\int_{\alpha+\frac{\pi}{3}}^{\frac{2\pi}{3}} V_m \sin(\omega t)\, d(\omega t) + \int_{\frac{\pi}{3}}^{\frac{2\pi}{3}+\alpha} V_m \sin(\omega t)\, d(\omega t) \right]$$

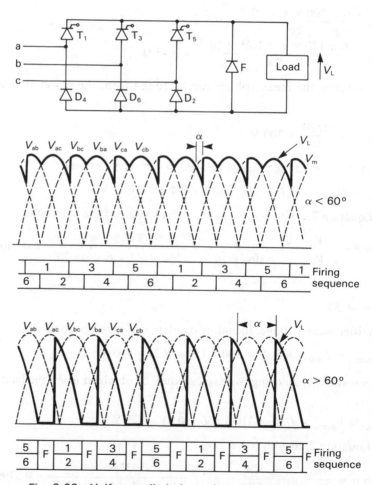

Fig. 2.22   Half controlled, three phase bridge converter.

$$= \frac{3}{2\pi} V_m (1 + \cos\alpha) \tag{2.24}$$

Overlap is ignored.

For firing angles $> 60°$, the commutating diode acts to prevent the reversal of the load voltage and commutates off the conducting thyristor and diode pair. The mean load voltage is now

$$V_{mean} = \frac{3}{2\pi} \int_\alpha^\pi V_m \sin(\omega t)\, d(\omega t)$$

Compare with Equation 2.24.

$$= \frac{3}{2\pi} V_m (1 + \cos\alpha) \tag{2.25}$$

Regulation

The effect of factors such as device voltage drops, device forward resistance, conductor resistance and the AC source inductance, in causing the converter output voltage on load (V_{load}) to differ from the ideal voltage (open circuit voltage V_{oc}, $I_L = 0$), is expressed by the regulation of the converter.

The open-circuit voltage (V_{oc}) is the ideal rectifier voltage with no overlap.

$$\text{Regulation} = \frac{V_{oc} - V_{load}}{V_{oc}} \times 100 \text{ per cent} \tag{2.26}$$

The voltage drop across the diodes and thyristors may be represented by a constant value, or more accurately as in Fig. 2.23, by a combination of a constant voltage and a resistance. The precise values used must take account of the firing angle.

The resistance of the leads and the AC source can be taken as constant in most systems. Where the bridge operation causes current to flow in two phases simultaneously then the effective AC source resistance in the equivalent circuit will be the sum of the phase resistances.

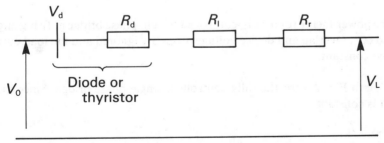

V_d = device voltage drop R_l = lead resistance
R_d = device resistance R_r = effective resistance due to overlap (voltage drop only)

Fig. 2.23   Rectifier equivalent circuit including device and lead components.

Power Factor

The general expression for power factor is:

$$\text{Power factor} = \frac{\frac{1}{T} \int_0^T vi\, dt}{V_{RMS}\, I_{RMS}} = \frac{\text{Mean power}}{V_{RMS}\, I_{RMS}} \qquad (2.27)$$

A converter has been shown to draw a non-sinusoidal current at supply frequency from the AC system and this current can therefore be represented by a fundamental component at the supply frequency and a series of harmonics. Assuming that the AC system voltage remains sinusoidal then power will be associated with only the fundamental frequency. Therefore

See Chapter 6.

$$\text{Power} = V_{1,RMS} I_{1,RMS} \cos \phi_1$$

$I_{1,RMS}$ and $V_{1,RMS}$ are the RMS amplitudes of the fundamental current and voltage; $\cos \phi_1$ is the phase displacement between $V_{1,RMS}$ and $V_{1,RMS}$.

$I_{RMS} = (I_{1,RMS}{}^2 + I_{2,RMS}{}^2 + I_{3,RMS}{}^2 + \dots)^{\frac{1}{2}}$
$V_{RMS} = V_{1,RMS}$ for an undistorted sinewave.

Substituting this relationship in Equation 2.27

$$\begin{aligned}
\text{Power factor} &= \frac{V_{1,RMS} I_{1,RMS} \cos \phi_1}{V_{1,RMS} I_{RMS}} \\
&= \frac{I_{RMS}}{I_{RMS}} \cos \phi_1 = \mu \cos \phi_1
\end{aligned} \qquad (2.28)$$

in which $\mu\ (= I_{1,RMS}/I_{RMS})$ is the current distortion factor.

Whenever harmonic currents are present then μ will be less than 1, even if the fundamental current and voltage are in phase ($\cos \phi_1 = 1$). For a fully-controlled converter with a constant load current and ignoring overlap then ϕ_1 will be equal to the firing angle α.

This means that a converter must be supplied with reactive volt-amperes (VARs) by the AC supply in order to operate. In the case of large converters this usually means that a VAR source is provided at the converter rather than relying on the capacity of the power system. Initially, this VAR source took the form of a rotary compensator but now more usually consists of a static compensator in which power semiconductor switches are used to switch in capacitors as required or to control a saturable reactor.

See Chapter 5 for case study of the Cross-Channel HVDC link.

Worked Example 2.6

Find the power factor for a fully-controlled, single-phase bridge at firing angles of 30° and 60°. Overlap and device voltage drops are ignored and the load current is assumed constant.

Referring to Fig. 2.3 for the fully controlled, single-phase bridge. Since the load current is constant

$$I_{RMS} = I_L$$

The mean load voltage is given by Equation 2.2

$$V_{mean} = \frac{2\sqrt{2}}{\pi} V_{RMS} \cos \alpha$$

The load power is then $V_{mean} I_L$ and

$$\text{Power factor} = \frac{2\sqrt{2}}{\pi} \cos \alpha$$

Since the load current is constant and overlap is ignored, $\cos \phi_1 = \cos \alpha$
Hence

$$\mu = I_{1,\text{RMS}}/I_{\text{RMS}} = \frac{2\sqrt{2}}{\pi} = 0.9003$$

and is independent of the firing angle

(i) $\alpha = 30°$
    Power factor = 0.7797

(ii) $\alpha = 60°$
    Power factor = 0.4502

Referring to Fig. 2.3 for the half-controlled bridge the thyristor current, and hence the supply current, is discontinuous. The RMS current is found from

$$I_{\text{RMS}} = \left[\frac{1}{\pi} \int_{\alpha}^{\pi} I_L^2 \, d\theta \right]^{\frac{1}{2}} = I_L \left[\frac{(\pi - \alpha)}{\pi}\right]^{\frac{1}{2}}$$

The mean load voltage is given by Equation 2.3

$$V_{\text{mean}} = \frac{1}{\pi} V_m (1 + \cos \alpha)$$

The mean load power is then $V_{\text{mean}} I_L$ and

$$\text{Power factor} = \frac{\sqrt{2}}{\pi} (1 + \cos \alpha) \left(\frac{\pi}{\pi - \alpha}\right)^{\frac{1}{2}}$$

The amplitude of the fundamental component of current is obtained from its Fourier coefficients as

See Appendix 2 for Fourier analysis.

$$b_1 = \frac{I_L}{\pi}\left[\int_{-(\pi-\alpha)}^{0} -\sin(\omega t) \, d(\omega t) + \int_{\alpha}^{\pi} \sin(\omega t) \, d(\omega t)\right]$$
$$= 2I_L (1 + \cos \alpha)/\pi$$

and

$$a_1 = \frac{I_L}{\pi}\left[\int_{-(\pi-\alpha)}^{0} -\cos(\omega t) \, d(\omega t) + \int_{\alpha}^{\pi} \cos(\omega t) \, d(\omega t)\right]$$
$$= 2I_L (\sin \alpha)/\pi$$

Amplitude of fundamental = $(a_1^2 + b_1^2)^{\frac{1}{2}} = 2\sqrt{2} I_L (1 + \cos \alpha)^{\frac{1}{2}}/\pi$.
RMS value of the fundamental is therefore $2I_L (1 + \cos \alpha)^{\frac{1}{2}}/\pi$
Hence

$$\mu = \frac{2}{\pi}\left(\frac{\pi}{\pi - \alpha}\right)^{\frac{1}{2}} (1 + \cos \alpha)^{\frac{1}{2}}$$

and

$$\cos \phi_1 = (1 + \cos \alpha)^{\frac{1}{2}}/\sqrt{2}$$

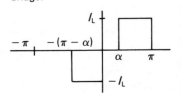

Supply current waveform for a two-phase, half-controlled bridge.

(i) $\alpha = 30°$
    Power factor = 0.9201
    $\mu = 0.9526$
    $\cos \phi_1 = 0.9659$

(ii) $\alpha = 60°$
    Power factor = 0.7397
    $\mu = 0.8541$
    $\cos \phi_1 = 0.866$

Transformer Rating

The need for special transformer winding configurations has been demonstrated already with various of the converter configurations. When selecting these transformers their rating under the particular operating conditions must be determined. This rating will in many cases be different for the primary and secondary windings. This may be contrasted with the conditions of normal transformer operation in which the rating will be the same for both windings.

The rating of any individual winding is obtained as the product of the RMS current through the winding and the RMS voltage across the winding.

Worked Example 2.7

A three-phase, half-wave, uncontrolled rectifier is supplying a constant current of 25 A at 240 V to its load. The rectifier is supplied from the secondary of an interconnected star transformer, the primary of which is connected to a three-phase, 660 V (line) supply. Find the ratings of the transformer primary and secondary windings.

From Equation 2.4 with $\alpha = 0°$

$$V_m = \frac{240 \times \sqrt{2} \times \pi}{3 \times \sqrt{2}} = 290.2 \text{ V}$$

Hence

$$V_{RMS} = V_m/\sqrt{2} = 205.2 \text{ V}$$

From Fig. 2.14 it can be seen that this voltage is obtained as the phasor sum of the voltages in each part of the secondary winding. These voltages are equal in magnitude (V_w) and differing in phase by 60°.

Hence

$$V_{RMS} = 3 \, V_w/\sqrt{2} = \sqrt{3} \, V_{w,RMS}$$

where $V_{w,RMS}$ is the RMS value of the voltage in each part of the secondary winding.

Thus

$$V_{w,RMS} = V_{RMS}/\sqrt{3} = 118.4 \text{ V}$$

As the current in each of the secondary windings flows for a third of a cycle

See Equation 2.5.

$$I_{2,RMS} = 25/\sqrt{3} = 14.43 \text{ A}$$

The primary winding voltage is obtained from the line voltage

$$V_{1,RMS} = 660/\sqrt{3} = 381 \text{ V}$$

The turns ration between the primary winding and its associated secondary windings is then

$$n = 381/118.4 = 3.218$$

The primary current flows for two-thirds of a cycle and has an amplitude of

$$I_1 = 25/3.218 = 7.77 \text{ A}$$

The RMS value of the primary current is obtained from

$$I_{1,\text{RMS}} = \left[\frac{1}{2\pi} \left(\int_{-\frac{2\pi}{3}}^{0} I_L^2 \, d\theta + \int_{\frac{\pi}{3}}^{0} I_L^2 \, d\theta \right) \right]^{\frac{1}{2}} = \frac{\sqrt{2}}{3} I_L = \frac{\sqrt{2} \times 7.77}{3}$$

$$= 6.34 \text{ A}$$

The ratings are then

Primary $= 3 \times 6.34 \times 381 = 7.25$ kW
Secondary $= 6 \times 14.43 \times 118.4 = 10.2$ kW

Converters with Discontinuous Current

Where the load inductance is insufficient to maintain the DC current at a constant value, the output current will contain a ripple component which will be reflected in the supply current, as in Fig. 2.24(a) and 2.24(b). Under light load conditions this current may well become discontinuous as in Fig. 2.24(c). Analysis of both converter and load behaviour is now much more complex and requires that individual component values be taken into account.

Arrillaga, J., Bradley, D.A. and Bodger, P.S. (1985). *Power System Harmonics.* John Wiley.

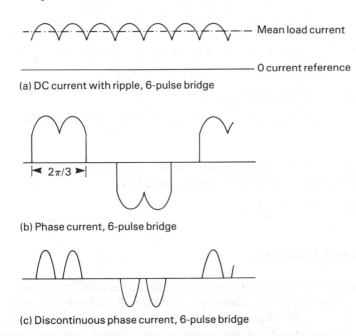

(a) DC current with ripple, 6-pulse bridge

(b) Phase current, 6-pulse bridge

(c) Discontinuous phase current, 6-pulse bridge

Fig. 2.24   Current waveforms for a 6-pulse bridge with a low inductance load.

The supply current will also be discontinuous when capacitive smoothing is used on the output of a rectifier as in Fig. 2.25(a). Here the diodes will start to conduct once the anode voltage exceeds that of the smoothing capacitor. Conduction ceases when the anode voltage falls below that of the capacitor. Figure 2.25(b) illustrates these conditions. As the load on the rectifier increases, the supply current will become more peaky in order to supply the energy requirements of the load as

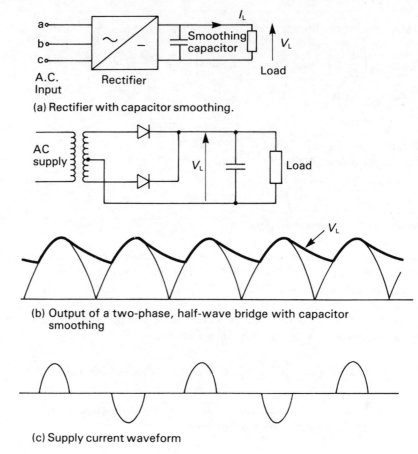

(a) Rectifier with capacitor smoothing.

(b) Output of a two-phase, half-wave bridge with capacitor
smoothing

(c) Supply current waveform

Fig. 2.25   Operation of a rectifier with capacitive smoothing.

shown by Fig. 2.25(c). Conduction still occurs over a part of each half cycle only
and the conduction period may be approximated by

$$\theta = 2\cos^{-1}(V_{mean}/V_{max}) \tag{2.29}$$

Converters with Voltage Bias

See Chapter 4 for a discussion
of DC machine operation.

Dewan, S.B., Slemon, G.R. and
Straughen, A. (1984). *Power
Semiconductor Drives*. John
Wiley.

When a converter is being used to supply a load such as a DC motor the back EMF
across the motor appears as a bias voltage on the DC side of the converter. The
operation of a single-phase, fully-controlled converter is then as shown in
Fig. 2.26. The performance of the converter under these conditions depends upon
the relationship between the firing angle (α) of the thyristors, the point (ψ) at which
the AC source voltage exceeds the bias voltage and the point (σ) at which the
thyristors stop conducting. Figures 2.26(b) to 2.26(d) illustrate one possible
condition for the operation of this converter with $\alpha > \psi$ and a discontinuous
current.

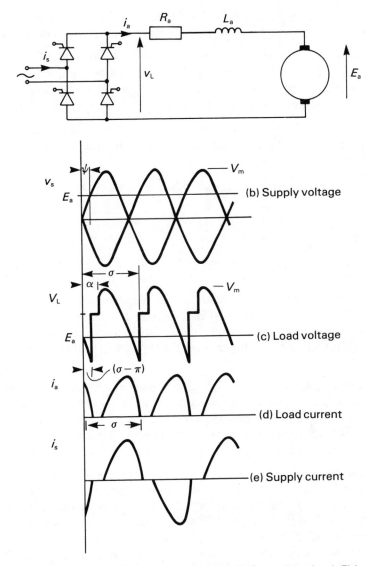

Fig. 2.26 Single phase controlled converter with D.C. machine load. Firing angle (α) greater than cut off angle (ψ) and ψ greater than $(0 - \pi)$.

Problems

2.1 A circuit such as that of Fig. 2.2(b) is supplied from a 50 Hz supply via a transformer such that:

$$V_{1,\text{RMS}} = V_{2,\text{RMS}} = 220 \text{ V}$$

Neglecting any voltage drop in the thyristors, find the mean load current at firing angles of 30° and 60° if the load is a pure resistance of 15 Ω. What will be the RMS and peak current in the thyristors under each of the above conditions?

If an inductance of 18 mH is included in series with the resistive load, estimate the firing angle at which the load current will become continuous.

2.2 A three-phase, half-wave converter is supplying a load with a continuous, constant current of 40 A over a range of firing angles from 0° to 75°. What will be the power dissipated by the load at these limiting values of firing angle? The supply voltage is 415 V (line).

2.3 A single-phase, half-controlled bridge is constructed as in the accompanying figure. Sketch the load voltage waveform for an inductive load at a firing angle of 60°.

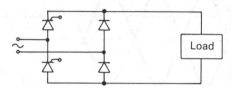

2.4 A half-controlled, single-phase bridge with a commutating diode as shown in Fig. 2.3(b) is fed by a 110 v, 50 Hz source and is supplying a constant load current of 20 A at a firing angle of 60°. If the source has an inductance of 0.34 H, find the overlap angles when the thyristor (a) turns on and (b) turns off.

2.5 A three-phase, fully-controlled bridge converter is fed from an inter-connected star transformer as in Fig. 2.14 and is supplying a highly inductive load of resistance 8 Ω. The transformer provides a secondary phase voltage of 240 V from a primary phase voltage of 660 V. Determine the rating of the transformer. Ignore overlap and thyristor volt drop.

2.6 A three-phase, fully-controlled bridge converter is supplying a DC load of 400 V, 60 A from a three-phase, 50 Hz, 660 V (line) supply. If the thyristors have a forward voltage drop of 1.2 V when conducting then, ignoring overlap, find (a) the firing angle of the thyristors, (b) the RMS current in the thyristors and (c) the mean power loss in the thyristors.
If the AC supply has an inductance per phase of 3.6 mH, what will be the new value of firing angle required to meet the load requirements?

2.7 A DC load with a maximum rating of 100 kV, 500 A is to be supplied by a twelve-pulse bridge converter made up of two bridge converters as in Fig. 2.21. Neglecting overlap and thyristor voltage drops, determine the required thyristor and transformer ratings for (a) parallel connection and (b) series connection of the bridges.

2.8 Obtain expressions for the variation of power factor with firing angle for (a) a fully-controlled, single-phase bridge and (b) a half-controlled, single-phase bridge supplying a constant load current.
Neglect overlap and device voltage drops.

2.9 A three-phase, fully-controlled bridge converter is connected to a three-phase, 50 Hz, 415 V (line) supply and is operating in the inverting mode at a firing advance angle of 30°. If the AC supply has a resistance and inductance per phase of 0.04 Ω and 1 mH respectively, find the DC source voltage, overlap angle and recovery angle when the DC current is constant at 52 A. The thyristors have a forward voltage drop when conducting of 1.8 V.

2.10 For the system of Problem 2.9, what will be the maximum DC current that can be accommodated at a firing advance angle of 22.5°, allowing for a recovery angle of 5°?

3 DC Choppers, Inverters and Cycloconverters

Objectives

☐ To examine the operation of thyristors with a DC source voltage.
☐ To introduce forced commutation and to consider the operation of various forced-commutation circuits.
☐ To consider the operation of a DC chopper.
☐ To classify DC choppers in terms of their operating envelopes.
☐ To examine the operation of voltage- and current-sourced converters as a means of producing a variable-frequency supply.
☐ To consider means of controlling a variable frequency inverter output voltage.
☐ To introduce pulse-width-modulated inverters.
☐ To introduce the cycloconverter.

Natural commutation.

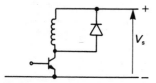

Freewheeling diode used to dissipate energy in inductive load on switching.

Chapter 2 described a range of circuits used to produce a DC voltage from an AC source voltage. In each of these circuits, the action of the AC source resulted in the conducting diode or thyristor being turned off at a natural current zero or on the transfer of load to another diode or thyristor.

Many applications such as variable-frequency inverters and chopper regulators operate from a DC source. Where power transistors, MOSFETs and GTO thyristors are used, turn-off can be achieved by control of the base or gate conditions. The ratings of these devices are, however, such that there remains a requirement to use thyristors to switch a DC source voltage. Thyristor turn-off under these conditions requires the use of external circuits and is referred to as *forced commutation*.

Forced Commutation Circuits

Silcon Controlled Rectifier Manual. General Electric, New York.

The function of a forced commutation circuit is to first reduce the current through the thyristor to zero and then to maintain a reverse voltage for a period equal to or greater than the thyristor turn-off time in order to re-establish the blocking state.

These objectives can be met by using an external voltage source to first reduce the current through the thyristor to zero by driving a reverse current of sufficient magnitude through the thyristor. The external voltage source then provides and maintains the required reverse voltage conditions across the thyristor to complete the turn-off. This can be achieved by using the arrangement of Fig. 3.1. The capacitor is charged initially in the direction shown on the figure then, when the switch is closed, the capacitor discharges, forcing a reverse current to flow through the thyristor, reducing the thyristor current to zero. The capacitor then continues to discharge through the load resistance, maintaining reverse voltage conditions across the thyristor during this period to complete the turn-off.

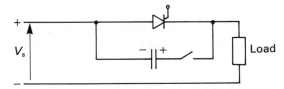

Fig. 3.1 Commutation by a parallel capacitor.

In practice, additional circuitry must be provided to control the charging of the capacitor and to initiate the discharge. Figure 3.2 shows a simple forced commutation circuit using a second thyristor to provide the control together with the associated current and voltage waveforms. At time t_0, the capacitor is charged as shown in the figure. When the commutating thyristor T_2 is fired at time t_1 the capacitor is connected across the main thyristor, T_1, forcing a reverse current and reducing the forward current to zero. The reverse voltage is then maintained across the thyristor until time t_2 at which point turn-off is complete. Thyristor T_2 will continue to conduct, charging capacitor C in the reverse direction via the load, turning off when the current falls below its holding level. This is the situation at time t_3. When thyristor T_1 is next fired, diode D starts to conduct, charging C in the original direction via the inductance L ready for the next commutation sequence to be initiated by firing T_2.

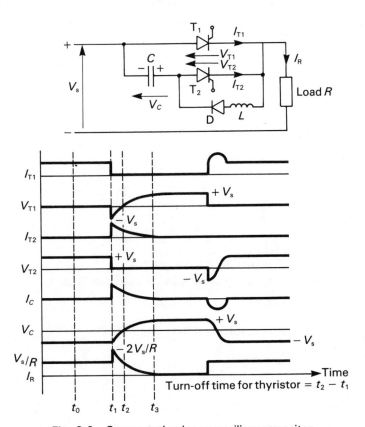

Fig. 3.2 Commutation by an auxiliary capacitor.

59

In the circuits of Figs 3.1 and 3.2, the thyristor is connected to the high-voltage side of the load and the gate circuit must therefore be fed from an isolated supply. Any of the methods considered in Chapter 1 for this purpose could be used.

Worked Example 3.1 The circuit of Fig. 3.2 is being used to supply a 12 Ω load from a 36 V source. The switching frequency is 250 Hz. Estimate the values of L and C and find the peak and RMS currents in thyristors T_1 and T_2 when the mean load voltage is at its minimum and maximum values. The thyristors each have a holding current of 50 mA and a turn-off time of 80 μs.

Turn-off of T_1 is complete when V_{T1} begins to go positive following the firing of T_2. From the curve of V_{T1} in Fig. 3.2:

$$v_1 = V_s (1 - 2e^{-t/RC})$$

when V_{T1} is zero

$$e^{-t/RC} = \tfrac{1}{2}$$
for $t = 80$ μs, $C = 9.62$ μF

Once the current in T_2 has fallen below the holding level, the reverse voltage across it must be maintained for 80 μs. From the curve of V_{T2} in Fig. 3.2 this period can be seen to be equal to a quarter cycle at a frequency of $1/[2\pi \sqrt{(LC)}]$. Therefore:

$$\frac{2\pi \sqrt{(LC)}}{4} = 80 \ \mu s$$

and

$$L = 0.27 \text{ mH}$$

Steady-state load current = 36/12 = 3 A
Peak value of the capacitor current is obtained from

$$\tfrac{1}{2}CV^2 = \tfrac{1}{2}LI^2$$

For a lossless system

$$I_{c,\text{max}} = V^2 \ \frac{C}{L} = 46.2 \text{ A}$$

which must be supplied by T_1.
   The peak current in T_1 is then 46.2 + 3 = 49.2 A
Peak current in T_2 is the capacitor current immediately on firing:

$$I_{T2,\text{max}} = 2V_s/R = 6 \text{ A}$$

T_2 stops conducting when the current falls to 50 mA.

$$\therefore \quad 50 \times 10^{-3} = 6e^{-t/RC}$$

and

$$t = 553 \ \mu s$$

which is the minimum off-time of T_1. T_1 may be fired before this, forcing T_2 off, but C will not be fully charged. Usually the off period is made long enough for C to have reached at least 80% of its maximum voltage.

The minimum on-time for T_1 is equivalent to a half cycle of the oscillatory waveform = 160 μs.

Minimum mean load voltage
RMS currents are found from:

$$I_{T1,RMS} = \left[\frac{1}{4 \times 10^{-3}} \int_0^{160 \times 10^{-6}} (3 + 46.2 \sin \omega t)^2 \, dt \right]^{\frac{1}{2}} = 7.08 \text{ A}$$

$$I_{T2,RMS} = \left[\frac{1}{4 \times 10^{-3}} \int_0^{553 \times 10^{-3}} (6e^{-t/RC})^2 \, dt \right]^{\frac{1}{2}} = 0.519 \text{ A}$$

Maximum mean load voltage
RMS currents are found from:

$$I_{T1,RMS} = \left\{ \frac{1}{4 \times 10^{-3}} \left[\int_0^{160 \times 10^{-6}} (3 + 46.2 \sin \omega t)^2 \, dt + \int_{160 \times 10^{-6}}^{3.467 \times 10^{-3}} 3^2 \, dt \right] \right\}^{\frac{1}{2}}$$

$$= 7.59 \text{ A}$$

$I_{T2,RMS}$ is as before.

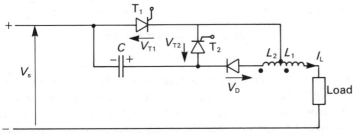

Fig. 3.3   Jones circuit.

The Jones circuit of Fig. 3.3 also uses an auxiliary thyristor for commutation purposes and has the advantage over the previous circuit of reliably initiating the commutation sequence from initial turn-on. This occurs since if the capacitor is initially discharged, then firing thyristor T_1 causes a voltage to be induced into inductance L_2 which charges C via diode D in the direction shown on the figure. Now when T_2 is fired the voltage on C appears across T_1 to turn it off.

Figure 3.4 shows two means by which an external voltage source can be used to turn off a conducting thyristor. In Fig. 3.4(a) a transistor switch is used to place the external voltage source across the conducting thyristor while in Fig. 3.4(b), a pulse transformer is used to introduce the commutating voltage into the main circuit.

The resonance set up in an LC circuit can be used directly to turn a thyristor off, eliminating the need for auxiliary thyristors and diodes. Figure 3.5(a) shows a simple series resonant turn-off circuit. Provided this circuit, including the load, is underdamped, then firing the thyristor will set up a current oscillation which will turn the thyristor off at the first current zero. The capacitor C will then discharge through the load. The on-time of the thyristor will be determined by the frequency of the oscillations.

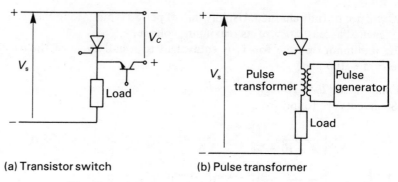

(a) Transistor switch   (b) Pulse transformer

Fig. 3.4   Commutation by an external source.

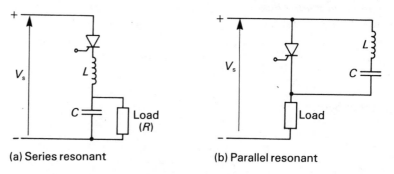

(a) Series resonant   (b) Parallel resonant

Fig. 3.5   Resonant turn-off.

Parallel resonance circuits such as that of Fig. 3.5(b) can also be used for thyristor turn off. In this circuit the capacitor C is charged during the thyristor off period to the supply voltage. When the thyristor is fired an oscillatory current is set up which, provided it is greater than the supply current, will turn the thyristor off. The thyristor ON period is again a function of the oscillatory frequency while the OFF period must be of sufficient duration to allow C to be adequately charged.

C is usually charged to at least 0.8 V_s

Bridge circuits

McMurray circuit.

Murphy, J.M.D. (1973). Thyristor Control of A.C. Motors. Pergamon, Oxford.

Assumes an inductive load, hence I_L is contant over the commutation interval.

More complex commutation circuits may be required when the thyristors are connected to form part of a bridge circuit. Figure 3.6 shows the configuration of one half of such a bridge circuit used to supply an inductive load.

In this circuit, T_1 and T_2 are the main thyristors making up the half-bridge and T_{1a} and T_{2a} are the auxiliary thyristors. Consider the conditions of Fig. 3.6 where T_1 is conducting with the capacitor C charged as shown. Firing T_{1a} at time t_0 allows C to discharge through the inductance L, producing an oscillatory current whose magnitude is arranged to be much greater than the load current. This current flows through T_1 in the reverse direction, reducing the current in T_1 to zero at time t_1, at which point diode D_1 diverts the excess current. The forward voltage of D_1 appears as a reverse voltage across T_1 during the period from time t_1 to t_2, completing the turn-off and re-establishing the blocking mode.

As the capacitor voltage reverses, the discharge current falls below the load

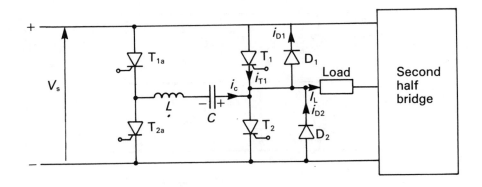

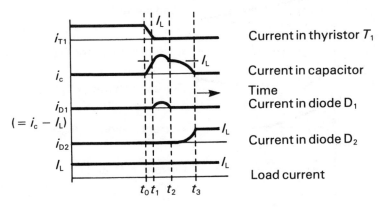

Fig. 3.6   McMurray circuit.

current and D_1 stops conducting at time t_2. The load current continues to flow via T_{1a}, charging C in the reverse direction to the source voltage at which point D_2 starts to conduct. D_2 then continues to take an increasing proportion of the load current as the energy in the magnetic field of L is transferred to the capacitor, reducing the current in T_{1a} to zero and turning it off to complete the commutation. Capacitor C is now charged to approximately $2V_s$ ready for the next commutation cycle with T_2 and T_{2a}.

The load current now decays to zero, turning D_2 off and allowing T_2 to start conducting, reversing the direction of current in the load. T_2 would normally be supplied with a continuous gate signal during this period to ensure turn-on at the appropriate instant.

A variation on this circuit is shown in Fig. 3.7. Initially, with T_1 conducting, capacitor C_1 is uncharged and C_2 is charged as shown. When T_2 is fired at time t_1 the bottom of inductor L_2 is connected to the supply negative. Since the capacitors cannot change voltage instantaneously the supply voltage V_s appears across L_2. As L_1 and L_2 are closely coupled an equal voltage is induced in L_1, raising the cathode potential of T_1 to $2V_s$ to turn T_1 off. The load current then transfers to T_2 and L_2, preserving the ampere-turns balance in the L_1L_2 coil and maintaining the reverse bias on T_1. The current in the inductive load is maintained during this period by the charging currents of capacitors C_1 and C_2. As C_2 discharges, the voltage across L_2 is decreased, reducing the voltage induced in L_1. At the same time C_1 is charging,

The opposite bridge is assumed to have been commutated simultaneously.

McMurray–Bedford circuit.

$L_1 = L_2 = L$ and $C_1 = C_2 = C$.

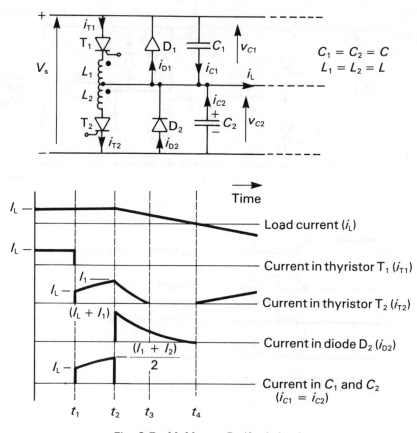

$C_1 = C_2 = C$
$L_1 = L_2 = L$

Fig. 3.7   McMurray-Bedford circuit.

eliminating the reverse bias on T_1 when the forward voltage on C_1 exceeds the reverse voltage on L_1.

The load current transfers to diode D_2 at time t_2, at which point C_1 is charged to V_s. The energy stored in L_2 is then dissipated in the loop L_2–T_2–D_2, with the current in T_2 falling to zero at time t_3. Diode D_2 continues to supply a decreasing current, turning off when the load current reaches zero at time t_4. A reverse load current can now be supplied via T_2.

Worked Example 3.2

A full bridge circuit using the commutation circuit of Fig. 3.6 is used to supply an inductive load such that load current is constant during commutation. The load resistance is 12 Ω and the bridge is supplied from a constant 400 V DC source. The thyristors used in the bridge have a turn-off time of 50 μs. Estimate component values for the circuit.

The reverse voltage, equal to the forward voltage drop of the parallel diode, appears across thyristor T_1 from time t_1 to t_2. Hence this must equal the turn-off time. From the waveform of capacitor current in Fig. 3.6 this period can be seen to correspond to that period for which I_c is greater than the load current. As I_c has the form:

$$i_c = I_{c,max} \sin \omega_0 t$$

where $\omega_0 = 1/\sqrt{(LC)}$

Then

$$I_L = I_{c,max} \sin \omega_0 t_1 \qquad\qquad \omega_0 t_1 < \pi/2$$

and

$$I_L = I_{c,max} \sin \omega_0 t_2 \qquad\qquad \omega_0 t_2 > \pi/2$$

Hence

$$\omega_0 t_2 - \omega_0 t_1 = \sin^{-1}(I_L/I_{c,max})$$

and

$$t_2 - t_1 = \text{turn-off time} = 50 \ \mu s$$

Energy available for turn-off $= \frac{1}{2}CV_c^2 = \frac{1}{2}LI_{c,max}^2$
Let $V_c = 2 \times 400 = 800$ V
Choosing $I_{c,max} = 1.5I_L$
Then

$$\omega_0 t_1 = 0.7297 \text{ and } \omega_0 t_2 = 2.4119$$

Thus

$$t_2 - t_1 = 1.6822/\omega_0$$

Therefore

$$\omega_0 = 1/\sqrt{(LC)} = 33643 \text{ rad s}^{-1}$$

Also, from energy relationship

$$C/L = I_{c,max}^2/V_c^2 = (1.5 \times 400/12)^2/800^2 = 3.906 \times 10^{-3}$$

and

$$C = 3.906 \times 10^{-3} L$$

Hence, from expression for ω_0

$$L = 0.476 \text{ mH and } C = 1.86 \ \mu F$$

DC Choppers

The DC chopper is used to provide a controllable DC output from a DC source by switching the source on to and off the load. By varying the switching frequency with a constant ON period or the mark–space ratio at constant frequency, the voltage at the load can be controlled.

Figure 3.8(a) shows a basic chopper regulator supplying an inductive load. The mean load voltage is

$$V_L = V_s t_1/T \tag{3.1}$$

while the RMS voltage at the load is given by

$$V_{L,RMS} = V_s\sqrt{(t_1/T)} \tag{3.2}$$

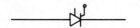
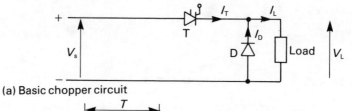

(a) Basic chopper circuit

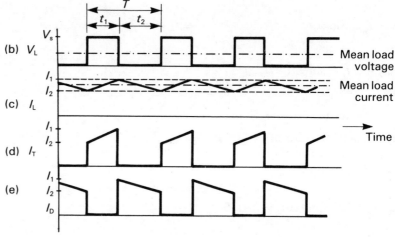

Fig. 3.8   Operation of a basic chopper with smoothing or T ≪ than system time constant.

Bird, B.M. and King, K.G.
(1983). *An Introduction to
Power Electronics*. John Wiley,
U.K.

With a switching rate and a load inductance such that the load current is continuous, the waveforms of current and voltage will be of the forms shown in Figs 3.8(b) and 3.8(c) respectively. If the period T is much less than the load time constant, or if a smoothing capacitor is used, the variation of the load current may be taken as being linear. Then, during conduction

$$V_s - V_L = L\,di/dt \equiv L\,\Delta i/\Delta t \tag{3.3}$$

and

$$I_1 - I_2 = (V_s - V_L)t_1/L \tag{3.4}$$

During the off period

$$I_1 - I_2 = V_L(T - t_1)/L = t_2 V_L/L \tag{3.5}$$

also

$$I_{mean} = (I_1 + I_2)/2 \tag{3.6}$$

Hence

$$I_1 = I_{mean} + t_2 V_L/(2L) \tag{3.7}$$

and

$$I_2 = I_{mean} - t_2 V_L/(2L) \tag{3.8}$$

The ripple current can then be expressed as

$$i_r = I_r\left(\frac{t}{t_1} - \frac{1}{2}\right) \qquad\qquad \text{for } 0 < t < t_1 \tag{3.9}$$

and

$$i_r = I_r \left(\frac{1}{2} - \frac{(t - t_1)}{t_2} \right) \qquad\qquad \text{for } t_1 < t < T \qquad\qquad (3.10)$$

where I_r is the peak-to-peak amplitude of the ripple current and

$$I_r = (I_1 - I_2)$$

The RMS value of the ripple current is then:

$$I_{r,\text{RMS}} = \left\{ \frac{1}{T} \left[\int_0^{t_1} I_r^2 \left(\frac{t}{t_1} - \frac{1}{2} \right)^2 dt + \int_{t_1}^{T} I_r^2 \left(\frac{1}{2} - \frac{(t - t_1)}{t_2} \right)^2 dt \right] \right\}^{\frac{1}{2}}$$
$$= (I_1 - I_2)/(2\sqrt{3}) \qquad\qquad (3.11)$$

If the period T is of the order of the system time constant then in the absence of smoothing the variation of current can no longer be considered as linear. With reference to Fig. 3.9

$$i_L = I_2 + \left(\frac{V_s}{R} - I_2 \right)(1 - e^{-Rt/L}) \qquad\qquad (3.12)$$

during conduction and

$$i_L = I_1 e^{-Rt/L} \qquad\qquad (3.13)$$

with the supply disconnected.

A further increase in T would result in the load current becoming discontinuous.

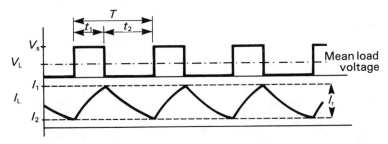

Fig. 3.9   Operation of a basic chopper with unsmoothed output where T is of the order of the system time constant.

Worked Example 3.3

A simple DC chopper is operating at a frequency of 2 kHz from a 96 V DC source to supply a load of resistance 8 Ω. The load time constant is 6 ms. If the mean load voltage is 57.6 V, find the mark–space ratio, the mean load current, the magnitude of the current ripple and its RMS value.

Period $= T = 1/f = 1/2000 = 0.5$ ms
Load time constant $= 12T$, therefore treat as a linear current variation.
From Equation 3.1

$$V_L = 57.6 = 96 t_1/T$$
$$\therefore \quad t_1 = 0.3 \text{ ms}$$

From Equation 3.2

$$V_{L,RMS} = 96 \times (0.3/0.5)^{1/2} = 74.36 \text{ V}$$

The mean load current = 57.6/8 = 7.2 A
From Equation 3.3

$$\text{Current ripple} = \Delta i = (V_s - V_L)\Delta t/L$$

Load time constant = L/R

$$\therefore \quad L = 6 \times 10^{-3} \times 8 = 48 \text{ mH}$$
$$\therefore \quad \Delta i = (96 - 57.6) \times 0.3 \times 10^{-3}/(48 \times 10^{-3}) = 0.24 \text{ A}$$

From Equation 3.7

$$I_1 = 7.2 + 57.6 \times 0.2 \times 10^{-3}/(2 \times 48 \times 10^{-3}) = 7.32 \text{ A}$$
$$\therefore \quad I_2 = 7.08 \text{ A}$$

From Equation 3.11

$$I_{RMS} = 0.24/(2\sqrt{3}) = 0.0693 \text{ A}$$

Dewan, S.B., Slemon, G.R. and Straughen, A. (1984). *Power Semiconductor Drives*. John Wiley, New York.

This basic circuit only allows power to flow from the supply to the load and is referred to as a class A or single-quadrant chopper as it operates only in the first quadrant of the $v_L - i_L$ diagram of Figs 3.10(a) or 3.10(b). Other chopper circuits capable of operating in one, two or four quadrants can be classified according to Fig. 3.10(c).

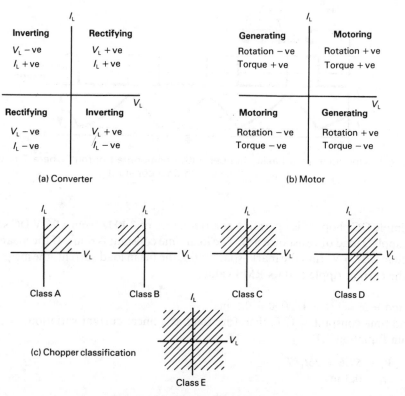

Fig. 3.10 Quadrant diagrams.

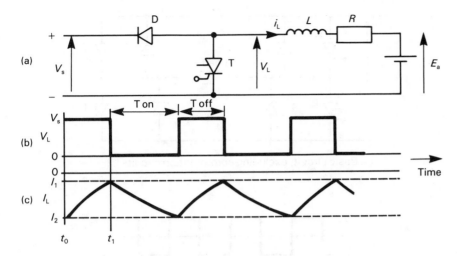

(a)

(b)

(c)

Fig. 3.11   Class B chopper.

Figure 3.11(a) shows a class B, step-up chopper. By turning on thyristor T, the load EMF E_a drives a current through inductor L. When T is commutated off, a proportion of the energy stored in L is returned to the supply via diode D. For the interval $0 < t < t_1$, D is conducting and

$$\frac{di_L}{dt} + \frac{R}{L} i_L = \frac{V_L - E_a}{L} \tag{3.14}$$

when, for the initial conditions of Figs 3.11(b) and 3.11(c)

$$i_L = \frac{V - E_a}{R}(1 - e^{-Rt/L}) + I_2 e^{-Rt/L} \tag{3.15}$$

When T is fired

$$\frac{di_L}{dt} + \frac{R}{L} i_L = -\frac{E_a}{L} \tag{3.16}$$

hence

$$i_L = -\frac{E_a}{L}(1 - e^{-Rt_x/L}) + I_1 e^{-Rt_x/L} \tag{3.17}$$

where $t_x = t - t_1$

Combining the circuits of Figs 3.8 and 3.11 gives the two-quadrant, class C chopper of Fig. 3.12. Care must be taken with this circuit to ensure that both thyristors T_1 and T_2 are not fired together as this would short-circuit the supply.

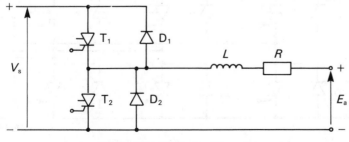

Fig. 3.12   Class C chopper.

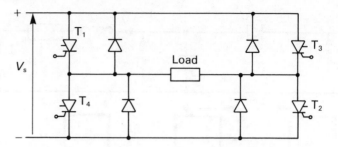

(a) Basic circuit, excluding commutation circuits

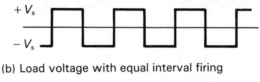

(b) Load voltage with equal interval firing

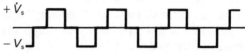

(c) Quasi-square wave output produced by delayed firing

Fig. 3.13 Voltage sourced, single phase bridge inverter.

Voltage-sourced Inverter

Compare this circuit with the McMurray and McMurray–Bedford circuits of Figs 3.6 and 3.7.

By combining two, two-quadrant choppers a full four-quadrant chopper can be produced. This is the basis of the voltage-sourced inverter, producing a bi-directional (alternating) current in the load. Figure 3.13(a) shows the basic circuit for a single-phase bridge inverter, excluding the necessary forced-commutation circuits. Reverse diodes are included in parallel with the thyristors in order to accommodate the phase relationship between current and voltage in inductive loads.

If the pairs of thyristors $T_1 - T_2$ and $T_3 - T_4$ are fired at equal intervals the load

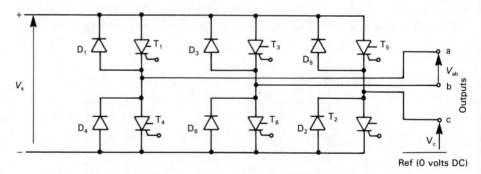

Fig. 3.14 Three phase bridge inverter.

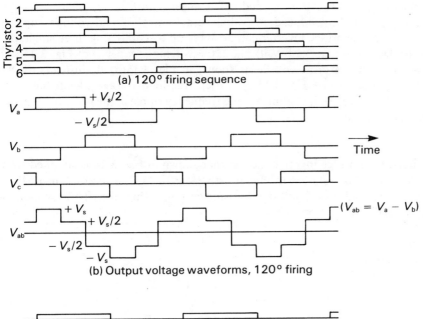

(a) 120° firing sequence

(b) Output voltage waveforms, 120° firing

$(V_{ab} = V_a - V_b)$

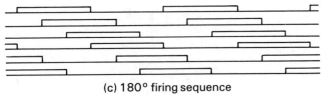

(c) 180° firing sequence

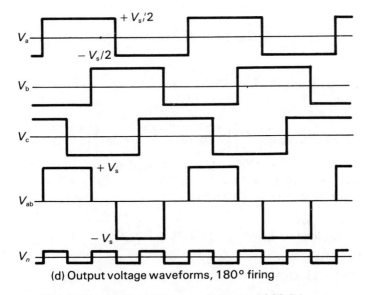

(d) Output voltage waveforms, 180° firing

Fig. 3.15   Output voltage waveforms, 180° firing.

voltage waveform will be a square wave as in Fig. 3.13(b). In applications such as induction-motor drives, some control of the amplitude of the load voltage is required. By delaying the firing of the appropriate pair of thyristors after the conducting pair have been turned off a quasi-square wave, such as shown in Fig. 3.13(c), can be produced, providing some control of load-voltage amplitude.

A three-phase bridge inverter can be made up by combining three single-phase half bridges as in Fig. 3.14. With the 120° switching sequence of Fig. 3.15(a) the load voltage waveforms will be as shown in Fig. 3.15(b). If instead, the 180° switching sequence of Fig. 3.15(c) is used, the load-voltage waveforms will be those of Fig. 3.15(d), including a triple frequency ripple in the neutral voltage of a star connected load.

Worked Example 3.4

A three-phase bridge inverter such as that shown in Fig. 3.14 is supplied from a 600 V source. For a star-connected resistive load of 15 Ω/phase find the RMS load current, the load power and the thyristor current ratings for (i) 120° conduction and (ii) 180° conduction.

Load is star connected.
(i) 120° conduction.

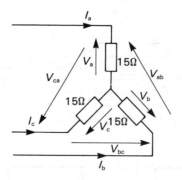

Example 3.4a   Star connected load.

Load current amplitude = $600/(2 \times 15) = 20$ A

$$\text{RMS load current} = \left\{\frac{1}{2\pi}\left[\int_0^{\frac{2\pi}{3}} 20^2 \, d\theta + \int_\pi^{\frac{5\pi}{6}} 20^2 \, d\theta\right]\right\}^{\frac{1}{2}}$$
$$= [(20^2 + 20^2)/3]^{\frac{1}{2}} = 16.33 \text{ A}$$

Load power = $16.33^2 \times 15 \times 3 = 12$ kW
Thyristor RMS current = $(20^2/3)^{\frac{1}{2}} = 11.5$ A

(ii) 180° conduction
At any instant, load on inverter = $15 + 15/2 = 22.5 \, \Omega$

$I_1 = V_s/22.5 = 600/22.5 = 26.67$ A
$I_2 = I_1/2 = 13.33$ A

Phases are connected in parallel for two-thirds of a cycle, therefore:

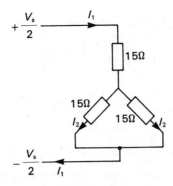

Example 3.4b   Effective load for 180° conduction.

$$\text{RMS load current} = \left\{ \frac{1}{2\pi} \left[\int_{0}^{\frac{2\pi}{3}} 13.33^2 \, d\theta + \int_{\frac{2\pi}{3}}^{\frac{2\pi}{3}} 26.67^2 \, d\theta + \int_{\frac{4\pi}{3}}^{2\pi} 13.33^2 \, d\theta \right] \right\}^{\frac{1}{2}}$$

$$= \left(\frac{2 \times 13.33^2 + 26.67^2}{3} \right)^{\frac{1}{2}} = 18.85 \text{ A}$$

Thyristors carry a current of 26.67 A for one-sixth of a cycle and 13.33 for a half cycle. Therefore the RMS current in a thyristor is:

RMS load current/2 = 13.33 A
Load power = $18.85^2 \times 15 \times 3 = 15.99$ kW

Figure 3.16 shows a single-phase, transformer-coupled inverter. By alternately firing and turning-off the thyristors the supply voltage is connected to each half of the transformer primary winding in turn, producing an alternating voltage in the secondary winding. The two halves of the primary winding must themselves be close coupled in order to transfer load current from one half of the primary to the other at turn-off of a thyristor. By combining two such inverters in series as in Fig. 3.17 then, by varying the relative firing instants, a quasi-squarewave output can be produced.

Also referred to as the bi-phase or centre-tapped inverter.

If transistors or GTO thyristors are used for the inverter instead of thyristors, the need for commutation circuitry is removed. Figure 3.18 shows a basic three-phase bridge inverter using transistors as the switching element. Inverters using

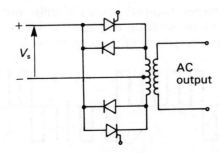

Fig. 3.16   Single phase, transformer coupled inverter.

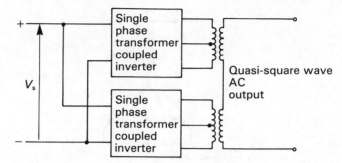

Fig. 3.17 Transformer coupled inverters connected in series to produce quasi square wave output.

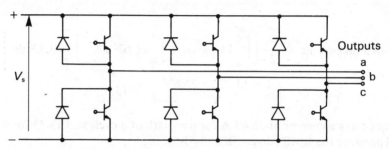

Fig. 3.18   Three phase transistor inverter.

transistors or GTO thyristors are capable of operating at much higher switching rates than inverters using conventional thyristors and therefore are used for high-frequency and pulse-width-modulated inverters.

Pulse-width-modulated Inverters

In the simplest form of pulse-width-modulated (PWM) inverter the supply voltage is switched at regular intervals to produce a load-voltage waveform such as that of Fig. 3.19. Control of the load voltage is achieved by varying the mark–space ratio of the pulses. By varying the pulse widths throughout the cycle an improvement in performance is obtained as the harmonic content of the output waveform is reduced. Emphasis is given usually to the reduction or elimination of the low-order harmonics since it is both easier and cheaper to filter the higher frequencies.

Figures 3.20 and 3.21 illustrate two approaches to the production of the pulse-width-modulated waveform based on the use of a combination of a reference sine-wave at the required output frequency and a triangular switching waveform. In each case, varying the amplitude of the reference sinewave varies the pulse widths and controls the effective amplitude of the output waveform.

Switching frequencies of 20 kHz or greater are used and switching loss becomes a major factor in a pulse-width-modulated inverter.

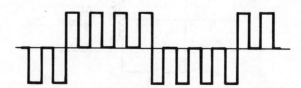

Fig. 3.19   Basic pulse width modulated waveform.

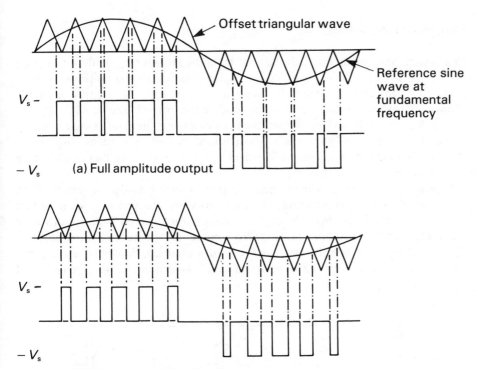

(a) Full amplitude output

(b) Reduced amplitude output

Fig. 3.20 Production of a pulse width modulated waveform using an offset triangular wave.

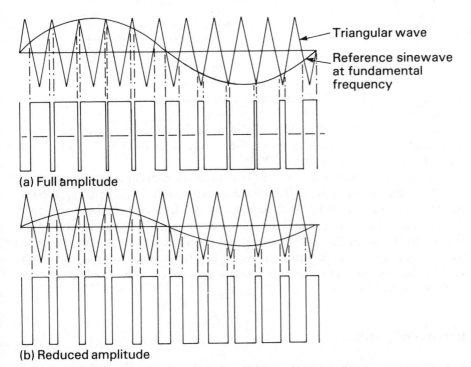

(a) Full amplitude

(b) Reduced amplitude

Fig. 3.21 Production of a pulse width modulated waveform using a triangular wave reference.

Current-sourced Inverter

In a current-sourced inverter, the current from the DC source is maintained at an effectively constant level, irrespective of load or inverter conditions. This is achieved by inserting a large inductance in series with the DC supply to enable changes of inverter voltage to be accommodated at low values of di/dt.

As it is a constant-current system, the current-sourced inverter is used typically to supply high-power-factor loads whose impedance either remains constant or decreases at harmonic frequencies in order to prevent problems either on switching or with harmonic overvoltages.

Figure 3.22 shows a single-phase, current-sourced bridge inverter. With thyristors T_1 and T_2 conducting, the capacitors are charged as shown. When thyristors T_3 and T_4 are fired the capacitors discharge through T_1 and T_2, turning them off. They will then continue to charge in the reverse direction via T_3-D_1-load-D_2-T_4. When the capacitors are fully charged, diodes D_3 and D_4 will start to conduct, reversing the load current which is eventually transfered to T_3 and T_4.

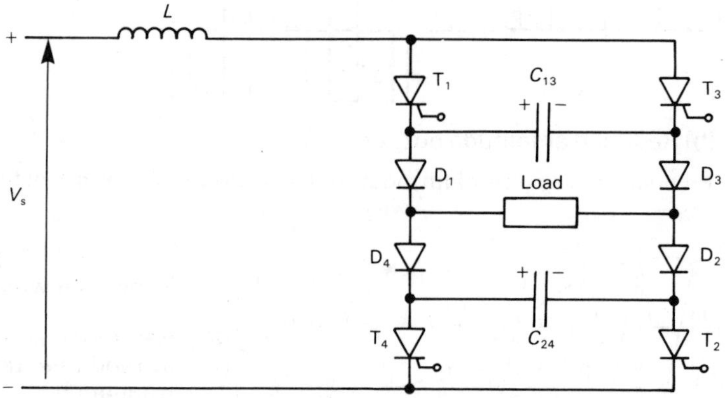

See the McMurray and McMurray–Bedford circuits considered earlier.

Fig. 3.22   Single phase, current sourced inverter.

This same commutation process is shown in the three-phase current-sourced inverter of Fig. 3.23. The thristors are fired in the order T_1-T_2-T_3-T_4-T_5-T_6-T_1, etc with each thyristor conducting for $120°$.

Commutation is performed by the commutating capacitors connected at the thyristor cathodes. Initially, C_{13} is charged as shown. When T_3 is fired, T_1 is reverse biased by C_{13} and turned off. With an inductive load, current continues to flow in the original direction via T_3 and D_1 until C_{13} is charged to V_{ba} when current begins to transfer to D_3. When this transfer of current is completed, commutation is ended and C_{35} is charged ready to turn T_3 off when T_5 is fired. Also, firing T_1 will turn T_3 via C_{13}. This means that the output phase sequence can be reversed without any additional circuitry.

The diodes have the additional function of isolating the capacitors from any load-voltage transients during commutation.

Inverter Performance

In addition to load-dependent losses in the switching devices a forced-commutated inverter suffers additional losses in the commutation circuit, in protection circuits

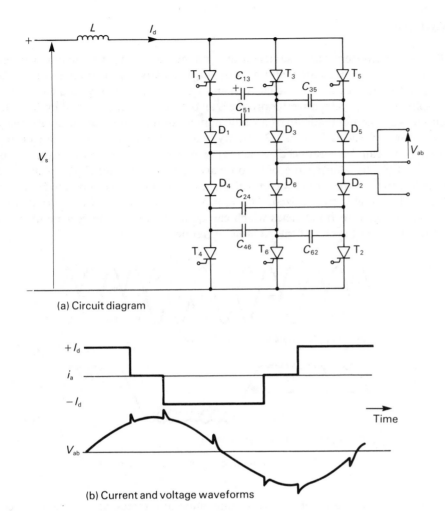

(a) Circuit diagram

(b) Current and voltage waveforms

Fig. 3.23   Three phase current sourced inverter.

such as the snubber circuits used to limit dV/dt and as switching losses in the devices. In a PWM inverter the switching losses will be relatively high, reducing overall efficiency and creating heat-removal problems.

Typical efficiencies are 96% for a quasi-squarewave inverter including the AC/DC converter and DC link, 91% for a PWM inverter using thyristors and 94% for a PWM inverter using transistors or GTO thyristors.

Quasi-squarewave inverters using thyristors normally operate over output frequencies from a few hertz to 100 Hz, or higher in special applications, with transistor inverters operating to 500 Hz. The PWM inverter tends to be limited by switching losses to output frequencies around 100 Hz with operation at higher frequencies in a quasi-squarewave mode.

Current-sourced inverters are typically operated over a frequency range from 5 to 50 Hz, the upper limit being set by the time required for commutation. Commutation losses are, however, small and the overall efficiency to the load is of the order of 96%.

Cycloconverters

Rissik, H. (1941). *Mercury-arc Current Converters*. Pitman, London.

Referred to as an envelope cycloconverter.

The cycloconverter synthesises its output voltage waveform by switching between the phases of the AC supply and provides an alternative to the inverter where the output frequencies are restricted to being less than the supply frequency. The simplest form of cycloconverter produces an output in which each half cycle of the output waveform is made up of a whole number of half-cycles of the single-phase supply waveform as in Fig. 3.24(a). By using a multi-phase supply an output waveform can be produced which approximates to a square wave as in Fig. 3.24(b). By altering the point-on-wave at which the individual phases are switched to form the output waveform, an output voltage can be obtained in which the fundamental is emphasized. This approach also means that the output is no longer restricted to frequencies which can be made up from integer numbers of cycles or parts of cycles of the AC source frequency.

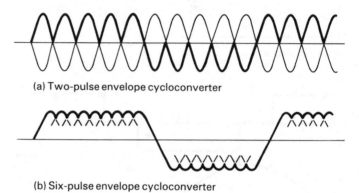

(a) Two-pulse envelope cycloconverter

(b) Six-pulse envelope cycloconverter

Fig. 3.24   Envelope cycloconverter waveforms.

The thyristors are naturally commutated.

Figure 3.25(a) shows the circuit for one phase of a three-pulse cycloconverter. From this figure it can be seen that if thyristors from the positive and negative groups were conducting simultaneously then the supply would be short-circuited. To avoid this possibility *blocked-group* or *inhibited-mode* operation is used, with the control circuitry arranged to prevent the simultaneous firing of thyristors in the positive and negative groups. The waveforms of Fig. 3.25(b) and 3.25(c) illustrate the operation of a blocked-group cycloconverter supplying a resistive and an inductive load respectively. In the latter case the effect of the inductance is to shift the phase of the load current with respect to the load voltage, taking each group into the inverting mode for part of each cycle. By increasing the pulse number of the cycloconverter a better approximation to a sinewave can be achieved at the output.

The peak output voltage that can be achieved is the peak DC voltage that each group can supply. Hence for a p-pulse cycloconverter and ignoring overlap:

$$V_{0,\text{max}} = \frac{p}{\pi} \sin\left(\frac{\pi}{p}\right) V_{\text{m}} \cos \alpha \tag{3.18}$$

The firing angle of the individual thyristors in the cycloconverter is determined by reference to the instantaneous value of output voltage required. The value of $\cos \alpha$,

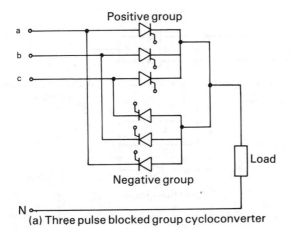

Positive group

a

b

c

Load

Negative group

(a) Three pulse blocked group cycloconverter

N

Each group operates alternately in the rectifying and inverting modes during each cycle.

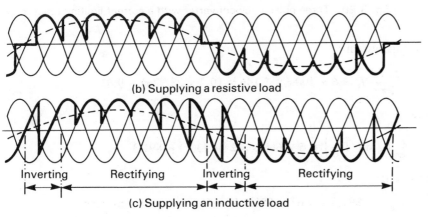

(b) Supplying a resistive load

Inverting   Rectifying   Inverting   Rectifying

(c) Supplying an inductive load

Fig. 3.25   Operation of a three pulse, blocked group cycloconverter.

and hence the firing angle (α), is then determined by reference to Equation 3.18.

As an alternative to blocked-group operation, a reactor can be connected as shown in Fig. 3.26, allowing both groups to conduct simultaneously as the reactor acts to limit any circulating current. This is the circulating current mode of operation of a cycloconverter. Cycloconverters require more complex control systems than other inverters which tends to limit their application to high-power systems with a variable frequency requirement below the supply frequency.

Worked Example 3.5

A six-pulse, blocked-group cycloconverter is fed from a three-phase, 600 V (line), 50 Hz supply. The supply has an inductance of 1.146 mH/phase. If the cycloconverter is supplying a variable resistive load with a current of 28 A, estimate the peak and RMS value of load voltage for firing angles of 0°, 30° and 60°.

The peak voltage is the mean voltage of the equivalent rectifier. Equation 2.21 gives

$$V_{mean} = \frac{p}{\pi} V_m \sin \left(\frac{\pi}{p} \right) \cos \alpha - \frac{p \omega L}{2\pi} I_L$$

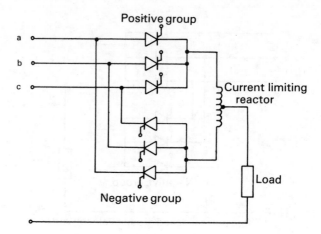

Fig. 3.26 Three pulse cycloconverter with a current limiting reactor.

For this system

$$\frac{p\omega L}{2\pi} I_L = 6 \times 100\pi \times 1.146 \times 10^{-3} \times 28/(2\pi) = 9.63$$

and

$$\frac{p}{\pi} V_m \sin\left(\frac{\pi}{p}\right) = 6 \times 660 \times \sqrt{2} \sin(30°) = 891.3$$

(i) $\alpha = 0°$

$V_{mean} = 891.3 - 9.63 = 881.7$ V $= V_{max}$ for cycloconverter

Hence the RMS voltage of the cycloconverter is

$V_{RMS} = V_{max}/\sqrt{2} = 623.4$ V

(ii) $\alpha = 30°$

$V_{mean} = 891.3 \cos(30°) - 9.63 = 762.3$ V $= V_{max}$ for cycloconverter

Hence the RMS voltage of the cycloconverter is

$V_{RMS} = V_{max}/\sqrt{2} = 539$ V

(iii) $\alpha = 60°$

$V_{mean} = 891.3 \cos(60°) - 9.63 = 436$ V $= V_{max}$ for cycloconverter

Hence the RMS voltage of the cycloconverter is

$V_{RMS} = V_{max}/\sqrt{2} = 308.3$ V

Problems

3.1 A series-resonant, forced-commutation circuit as in Fig. 3.5(a) has values of 2.8 mH and 24 μF. The load resistance is 40 Ω. If the DC source voltage is

120 V, find the mean power in the load if the thyristor is being fired at (a) 250 Hz and (b) 500 Hz.
[Note: This is a problem which requires a numerical solution.]

3.2 An ideal DC chopper operating at a frequency of 600 Hz supplies a load of resistance 5 Ω, inductance 9 mH from a 110 V DC source. If the source has zero impedance and the load is shunted by an ideal diode as shown, calculate the mean load voltage and current at mark/space (on/off) ratios of (a) 1/1; (b) 5/1; and (c) 1/3.

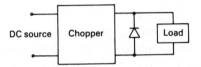

3.3 A single-phase bridge inverter using the McMurray–Bedford commutation circuit of Fig. 3.7 is being used to supply a load of 8 Ω resistance from a 300 V DC source. If the load inductance is such that the current remains constant over the commutation interval, estimate the component values for a thyristor turn-off time of 50 μs. Assume components are ideal.

(Hints: (i) The oscillation involves a total stored energy of $\frac{1}{2}CV_s^2 + \frac{1}{2}L\,I_L^2$ at a frequency of $1/(2\pi\sqrt{2LC})$.

   (ii) The time required for turn-off is the time taken for the capacitor voltage to fall to half its initial value.

   (iii) The current in the inductor has the form $i_c = I_m \sin(\omega t + \phi) - I_L$. Assume that I_m has a value of 2.6 times the steady-state load current.

   (iv) Charge lost by C_2 equals charge gained by C_1.

   (v) The additional stored energy in the inductor is supplied by the source.)

3.4 A single-phase bridge inverter such as that of Fig. 3.13 is used to supply a load of 10 Ω resistance, 24 mH inductance from a 360 V DC source. If the inverter is operating at 60 Hz, determine the steady-state power delivered to the load for (a) squarewave operation; (b) quasi-squarewave operation with an 'on' period of 0.6 of a cycle.

3.5 A single-phase, current-sourced inverter such as shown in Fig. 3.22 is used to supply a resistive load of 16 Ω from a 200 V DC source. If the thyristors have a turn-off time of 40 μs and the inverter output frequency is 40 Hz, estimate suitable values for the source inductance and commutating capacitors. Neglect all device voltage drops and losses and assume a maximum di/dt value of 16 A/s.

3.6 A three-pulse cycloconverter is supplying a single-phase load of 480 V, 72 A at a power factor of 0.85 lagging and a frequency of 25 Hz. Estimate the minimum supply voltage required, the ratings of the thyristors and the power factor of the AC supply. Neglect losses and device voltage drops.

4 Applications I — Drives

Ward-Leonard, H. (1896). Volts versus ohms — the speed regulation of electric motors. *AIEE Transactions*, **13**, 375–84.

Objectives

☐ To introduce basic principles of DC and AC induction machines.
☐ To consider their operation in the motoring, generating and braking modes.
☐ To introduce the principles of variable-speed drives as applied to both DC and AC induction machines.
☐ To examine means of control.
☐ To compare analogue and digital control systems.
☐ To consider some applications of variable speed drives.
☐ To consider briefly other types of electric motor.

Many industrial applications require the provision of a variable-speed rotary drive for their operation. In 1896 Harry Ward-Leonard laid down the basis of an effective and efficient means of controlling DC motors which endured until the development of power electronic drives from the 1960s onwards. Indeed, many of the principles of his original system are still to be found in current variable-speed drive technology.

Ward-Leonard drive; DC generator is used to provide a variable voltage supply for a DC motor.

Initially the majority of variable-speed drives used DC motors as the work machine because the provision of the variable-frequency supply required to control an AC machine was complicated and uneconomic. However, the development of controllable power electronic switching devices has resulted in the development of a wide range of drives using both DC and AC induction motors. More recently, microprocessor-based digital control systems have replaced the analogue controllers, giving an increased sophistication of operation and facilitating the use of machines such as stepper motors and the switched reluctance motor.

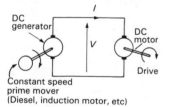

DC Machines

The DC machine consists of the stationary field winding and a rotating armature winding as shown in Fig. 4.1. The field winding is supplied with a DC current to

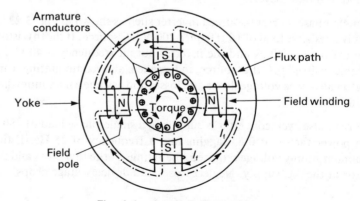

Fig. 4.1 4-pole D.C. machine.

produce a static magnetic field pattern within the machine. This magnetic field then interacts with the current in the armature conductors to produce a torque. In order to sustain this torque the armature current distribution must be maintained relative to the field, irrespective of the actual rotor position. This is achieved by the action of the commutator which reverses the current in the armature conductors as they pass from under one field pole to the next. Also, as the armature conductors are moving through the magnetic field produced by the field winding they have induced in them a back EMF (E_a) which appears at the commutator.

When motoring, the DC machine draws power from the DC source and the torque developed by the machine acts to rotate the armature against the applied mechanical load. In the generating mode, the torque developed opposes the applied mechanical torque driving the armature. The defining steady state equations are, with reference to Fig. 4.2:

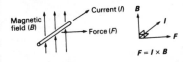

The force on a conductor in a magnetic field is given by

$F = I \times B$

The commutator acts as a mechanical rectifier.

Induced voltage is a function of field strength and conductor velocity.

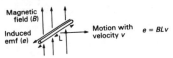

$e = BLv$

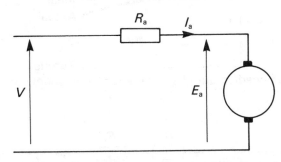

Fig. 4.2   D.C. machine armature circuit (motoring).

Generating	$E_a = V + I_a R_a$	(4.1)
Motoring	$E_a = V - I_a R_a$	(4.2)
	$E_a = K\phi\omega$	(4.3)

where ϕ = Flux per pole
and ω = Rotational speed in radians per second.

$$\text{Internal mechanical power} = T\omega = E_a I_a \qquad (4.4)$$

Therefore

$$\text{Torque} = T = K\phi I_a \qquad (4.5)$$

Equation 4.4 takes no account of mechanical losses such as windage and friction. Useful mechanical power output = Internal mechanical power minus mechanical losses.

The field winding can either be supplied from a separate DC source (shunt connection) or be connected as part of the armature circuit (series connection). Figure 4.3 shows these connections together with the motoring torque/speed characteristics that result.

K is a constant determined by the physical parameters of the machine.

Motoring

Neglecting armature resistance then, from equations 4.2 and 4.4

$$V = E_a = K\phi\omega \qquad (4.6)$$

If V is held constant it can be seen from Equation 4.6 that the motor speed (ω) can be controlled by varying the field (ϕ) such that

Field control.

$$\omega \propto 1/\phi \qquad (4.7)$$

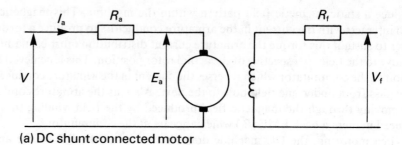

(a) DC shunt connected motor

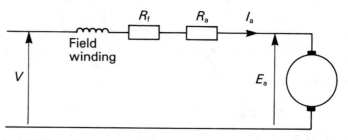

(b) Speed/torque characteristic of a DC shunt motor

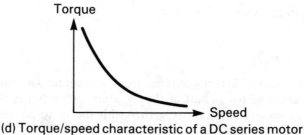

(c) DC series connected motor

(d) Torque/speed characteristic of a DC series motor

Fig. 4.3   D.C. motor connections and characteristics.

The maximum continuous armature current is the rated current for the machine.

For a constant power. Torque ∝ 1/ω.

The limiting condition for maximum speed is set mainly

The limiting condition for continuous operation is the maximum continuous current that can be carried by the armature winding. Using Equations 4.4 and 4.6 with V (and hence E_a) constant, the machine is seen to operate with a constant power limit. This condition is shown by Fig. 4.4. The minimum speed obtainable using field control occurs at conditions of maximum applied armature voltage and maximum field. Speed can be varied over a range of about 2 to 1 for large machines and 4 or 5 to 1 for small machines.

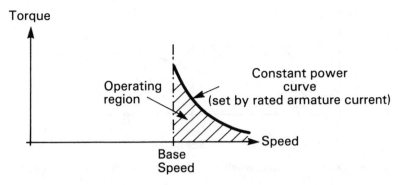

Fig. 4.4   Operating region of a D.C. motor with field control.

Referring again to Equation 4.6, if the field (ϕ) is held constant then the motor speed can be controlled by varying the voltage applied to the machine armature when

$$V \propto \omega \tag{4.8}$$

Applying the same restriction on armature current as before, then, by reference to Equation 4.3 the motor is found to operate with a constant torque limit as in Fig. 4.5. The maximum operating speed occurs with maximum armature voltage and maximum field with an operating speed range of the order of 100 to 1. Figures 4.4 and 4.5 can now be combined to give the full operating envelope of Fig. 4.6.

by commutation behaviour under weak field conditions.

Armature voltage control.

These are the same conditions that define the minimum speed conditions with field control.

A separately excited 220 V DC shunt motor is rated at 1.5 kW at 900 r/min when the armature current is 8.2 A. Armature resistance is 2.4 Ω. Mechanical losses can be represented by a torque which varies directly with motor speed.

Worked Example 4.1

With the field current set at the value required to give rated speed at rated load and armature voltage, find the values of armature voltage required and the armature current when the motor is operating against a load torque of 3.5 Nm at rated speed.

For operation at rated speed and load:

Input power to motor $= VI_a = 220 \times 8.2 = 1804$ W
$I_a^2 R_a$ loss $= 161.4$ W
Rotational losses $=$ Input power $-$ Output power $- I_a^2 R_a$ loss
$\qquad\qquad = 1804 - 1500 - 161.4 = 142.6$ W

For constant torque power $\alpha \omega$.

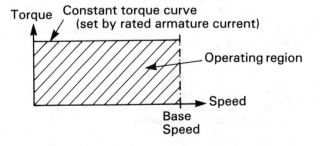

Fig. 4.5   Operating region of a D.C. motor with armature voltage control.

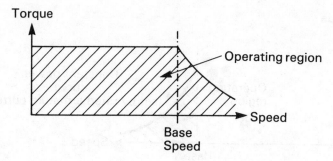

Fig. 4.6   Operating region combining field and armature voltage control.

Mechanical loss torque $= 142.6/(2\pi \times 900/60) = 1.51$ Nm
$E_a = V - I_aR_a = 220 - 8.2 \times 2.4 = 200.3$ V

From $E_a = K\phi\omega$

$K\phi = 200.3/(2\pi \times 900/60) = 2.125$

When operating against a 3.5 Nm load torque at rated speed the total torque developed by the motor is

Motor torque $= 3.5 +$ Mechanical loss torque $= 5.01$ Nm

Now Torque $= T = K\phi I_a$

$\therefore\quad I_a = T/K\phi 5.01/2.125 = 2.36$ A

and

$$V = E_a + I_aR_a = K\phi\omega + I_aR_a = 2.125 \times 2\pi \times 900/60 + 2.36 \times 2.4$$
$$= 205.9 \text{ V}$$

Braking

During variable-speed operation the motor will be required to both accelerate and decelerate. The deceleration process can be assisted where required by the various forms of electrical braking shown in Fig. 4.7. In Fig. 4.7(a) the armature is

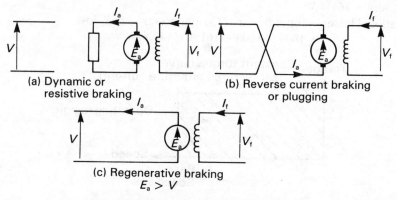

Fig. 4.7   D.C. machine braking modes.

disconnected from the supply and connected to a resistor. With the field applied, an EMF is produced which drives a current through the resistor, dissipating the energy stored in the rotating inertia of the armature.

Resistive or dynamic braking.

By reversing the connection of the armature to the supply, as in Fig. 4.7(b), the direction of current through the armature is reversed. This produces a reverse torque which rapidly decelerates the motor. Since the machine equation has the form under these conditions of

Plugging. This is a very severe operating condition.

$$-V = E_a + I_a R_a \tag{4.9}$$

a current-limiting resistor would normally be included to control the armature current. If the field is adjusted to make $E_a > V$ the machine will act as a generator returning energy from the mechanical system to the DC supply as in Fig. 4.7(c). The maximum field is limited by the field voltage supply and the maximum permitted field current.

Regenerative braking.

DC Machine Dynamics

Consideration thus far has been in terms of steady-state conditions. In practice many operating conditions involve the dynamic behaviour of the machine. Such cases require the effects of the machine armature and field inductances, the rotary inertia and the non-linearities of the magnetic circuit to be taken into account. The machine equations are re-written as:

Lower case is used to represent instantaneous values.

$$v = e_a \pm (i_a R_a + L_a di_a/dt) \tag{4.10}$$
$$T = K\phi i_a = T_L + Jd\omega/dt \tag{4.11}$$

+Motoring; −Generating.

where T_L is the load torque
J is the rotary inertia and L_a is the armature inductance

$$e_{a.} = K\phi\omega \tag{4.12}$$

For the field circuit

$$v_f = i_f R_f + L_f di_f/dt \tag{4.13}$$
$$\phi = f(i_f) \tag{4.14}$$

The relationship between ϕ and i_f is non-linear and is a function of the magnetic properties of the materials used.

where L_f is the field circuit inductance.

A separately excited DC motor is operating from a fully controlled bridge under light load conditions such that the current and voltage waveforms are as shown in the margin. Find an expression for the armature current and hence find expressions for the mean values of armature current and armature voltage in terms of firing angle.

Worked Example 4.2

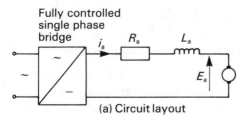

Fully controlled
single phase
bridge

(a) Circuit layout

Example 4.2   (See also Fig. 2.26).

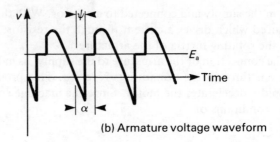

(b) Armature voltage waveform

Example 4.2   cont'd

When the thyristors are fired at $\omega t = \alpha$

$$v - e_a = i_a R_a + L_a(di_a/dt)$$

Assuming e_a constant at E_a

$$V_m \sin(\omega t) - E_a = i_a R_a + L_a(di_a/dt)$$

Let $\omega t = \omega \tau + \alpha$
Using Laplace Transforms

$$V_m \left(\frac{\omega \cos \alpha}{s^2 + \omega^2} + \frac{s \sin \alpha}{s^2 + \omega^2} \right) - \frac{E_a}{s} = I_a(s)R_a + sL_a I_a(s)$$

Solving

$$i_a = \frac{V_m}{Z} [\sin(\omega \tau + \alpha - \phi) + \sin(\phi - \alpha)e^{-\gamma \tau}] - \frac{E_a}{R_a} (1 - e^{-\gamma \tau})$$

Substituting for τ

$$i_a = \frac{V_m}{Z} [\sin(\omega t - \phi) + \sin(\phi - \alpha)e^{-\gamma(\omega t - \alpha)/\omega}] - \frac{E_a}{R_a} [1 - e^{-\gamma(\omega t - \alpha)/\omega}]$$

where

$$Z = (R_a^2 + L_a^2)^{1/2}$$
$$\gamma = R_a/L_a$$

If conduction ceases at an angle ψ, the mean current is given by

$$I_a = \frac{1}{\pi} \int_\alpha^\psi i_a \, dt$$

$$= \frac{1}{\pi} \left\{ \frac{V_m}{Z} \left[\cos(\alpha - \phi) - \cos(\psi - \phi) \right] - \frac{E_a}{R_a} (\psi - \alpha) + \frac{\omega}{\gamma} \left[\frac{V_m}{Z} \sin(\phi - \alpha) + \frac{E_a}{R_a} \right] (1 - e^{-\gamma(\psi - \alpha)/\omega}) \right\}$$

The load voltage is made up of three components:

$$v_L = -V_m \sin \omega t \qquad\qquad 0 < \omega t < (\psi - \pi)$$
$$v_L = E_a \qquad\qquad (\psi - \pi) < \omega t < \alpha$$
$$v_L = V_m \sin \omega t \qquad\qquad \alpha < \omega t < \pi$$

Therefore

$$v_L = \frac{1}{\pi}\left[\int_0^{\psi-\pi} -V_m \sin(\omega t)\, d(\omega t) + \int_{\psi-\pi}^{\alpha} E_a\, d(\omega t) + \int_{\alpha}^{\pi} V_m \sin(\omega t)\, d(\omega t)\right]$$

$$= \frac{1}{\pi}[V_m(\cos\alpha - \cos\psi) + E_a(\alpha + \pi - \psi)]$$

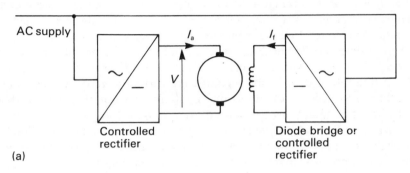

Controlled rectifier

Diode bridge or controlled rectifier

(a)

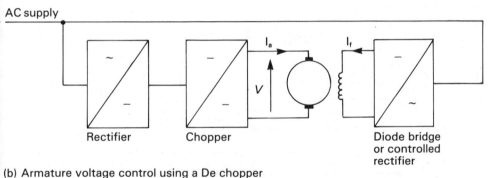

Rectifier

Chopper

Diode bridge or controlled rectifier

(b) Armature voltage control using a De chopper

Fig. 4.8   Variable speed drives using armature voltage control.

Variable-speed DC Drives

The most common form of variable-speed DC drive is based on the control of armature voltage. Figure 4.8(a) shows a simple system using a controlled rectifier which must be of the fully controlled type if regeneration is required. An alternative is to use a diode rectifier to supply a DC chopper as in Fig. 4.8(b). A chopper would be used also where a DC supply is already available.

The speed of the motor is set by the mean armature voltage with any torque oscillations being damped out by the smoothing action of the system inertia.

For large motors (>2.5 kW) the armature inductance is normally sufficient to maintain a constant DC current under all but very light load conditions. Whatever the size of motor, it is derated to some extent by virtue of the presence of harmonics in the motor supply, since these do not produce any useful mechanical torque but increase the electrical and magnetic losses in the machine. This derating is less the larger the machine as the increasing inductance smooths out current variations. In particular, DC machines intended specifically for use with thyristor converters are

Uncontrolled converter. Operation in first quadrant. See chapter 3.

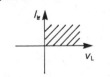

Controlled converter. Two quadrant operation.

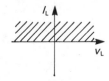

designed with laminated field poles and have an increased armature inductance to give an armature phase angle of the order of 75° to 85°.

Reversing Drives

The direction of rotation of a DC machine can be reversed by reversing either the armature voltage or the field, using any of the arrangements shown in Fig. 4.9. If half-controlled converters are used with contactor reversal (Fig. 4.9(a)) or for the dual bridge arrangement (Fig. 4.9(b)), the machine is first brought to rest and the armature current reduced to zero. Once at rest the second bridge is switched on or the contactor reversed to drive the motor in the reverse direction.

Where fully-controlled bridges are used, full four-quadrant operation can be obtained. When used with contactor reversal the firing angle of the conducting bridge is first retarded, reducing the armature current to zero. At this point the contactor is reversed. As the direction of rotation has not altered from that of Fig. 4.10(c), the conditions are now those of Fig. 4.10(b) with the converter operating in the inverting mode and regenerative braking taking place. The firing angle of the converter is now advanced until at zero speed it reverts to the rectifying mode and the motor is driven in the reverse direction (Fig. 4.10(c)).

Operation in both motoring quadrants.

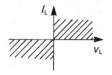

Full 4-quadrant operation.

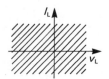

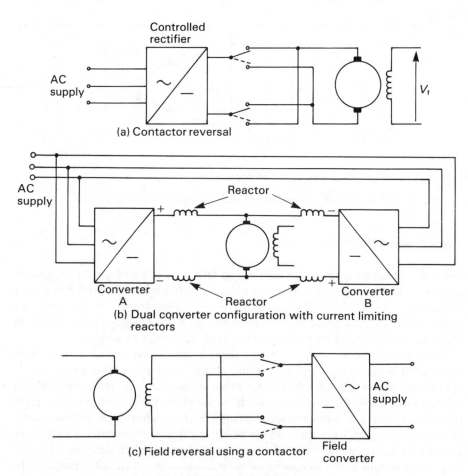

(a) Contactor reversal

(b) Dual converter configuration with current limiting reactors

(c) Field reversal using a contactor

Fig. 4.9   Reversing drives.

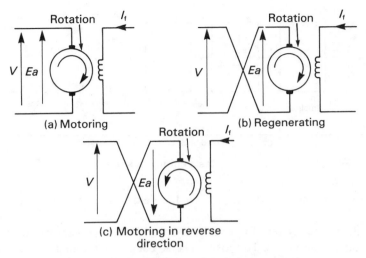

Fig. 4.10 Operating modes during reversal.

Operation of the contactor can introduce a delay of around 0.2 s over which period no torque is developed. While this may be acceptable for drives such as presses, hoists, lathes and marine propulsion where reversals are infrequent, there are other applications, as for example steel strip mills and paper mills, where a more rapid reversal is required. This can be achieved by using the dual bridge arrangement of Fig. 4.9(b). During reversal the two bridges are controlled so as to have the same mean output voltages. As the instantaneous voltages cannot, however, be the same, reactors are included to limit the circulating current. Alternatively, the bridges may be controlled so that only one bridge is conducting at any instant. This permits the removal of the reactors but at the expense of an increase of around 10 ms in the time required for torque reversal.

Field reversal can also be achieved by means of dual bridges or contactors. The reversal of the field current is relatively slow because of the need to remove the stored energy of the field prior to current reversal and this introduces delays of about 1 s into torque reversal. Field forcing, in which a high initial voltage is applied to the field, is used to produce a rapid initial rise of current to speed up the reversal. The field voltage is then reduced to the value required to maintain the desired field current.

Control

A drive control system may be required to perform a combination of functions including:

(a) Responding to changes in demand speed or torque.
(b) To provide start-up and shut-down procedures.
(c) To ensure that operation is largely independent of fluctuations in supply conditions.
(d) To optimize the operating conditions for best performance.

The control system may also be required to provide protection against overloads and faults, to maintain a check on drive status and performance, to synchronize the

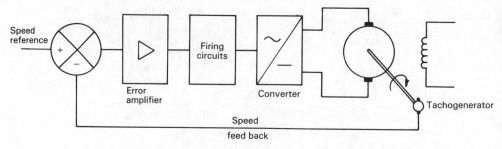

Fig. 4.11   Basic control system.

operation of a number of drives, to provide field forcing and operate reversing drives.

The basic control system for a variable-speed DC drive is shown in Fig. 4.11. Information on output speed or position is fed back to the comparator, the output of which is used to control the operation of the converter. Because of the low armature resistance of the motor, such a system, with changes of demand load or speed, could result in excessive currents being drawn from the supply. Some means of limiting current is therefore included as part of the control system.

Figure 4.12 shows a typical speed control system for a single-quadrant drive. The set speed is fed to the comparator via a ramp generator to smooth out the effect of sudden changes. There it is compared with the speed reference derived from a tachogenerator on the output shaft. The comparator error signal is then taken to an output limited amplifier which restricts the maximum error signal and hence the maximum current. This error signal is then compared with the motor current which may be obtained either by means of a direct current current transformer (DCCT) or an AC current transformer and rectifier in the converter supply lines. The output of this second comparator is then used to control the firing angle of the converter.

The converter is effectively acting as a power amplifier.

See Chapter 5, Fig. 5.4, etc. for discussion of the Direct Current Transformer.

PID controller = *P*roportional, *I*ntegral and *D*erivative controller. Also referred to as a Three Term controller.

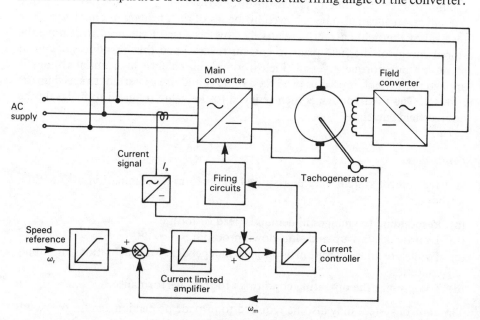

Fig. 4.12   Speed controller.

In the form shown, the controller will operate with a speed error. This could be eliminated by modifying the controller to incorporate a full PID control scheme.

Analogue controllers of the type described can provide a speed stability of about 0.1%. Recently, control systems based on microprocessors and offering greater precision, flexibility, consistency, stability and noise immunity have largely replaced analogue systems. By using digital techniques the speed stability can be improved to around 0.01%. In addition, digital systems enable precise speed matching or controlled speed ratios between two or more motors by the use of a common speed reference. Such a system can also enable the phase relationship between the drive shafts of a number of motors to be controlled.

The electronic gearbox.

Case Study — Servo Amplifier, Renold plc

DC servomotors are used to provide the drive for a range of motions. The configuration of a typical servomotor drive is shown in schematic form by Fig. 4.13.

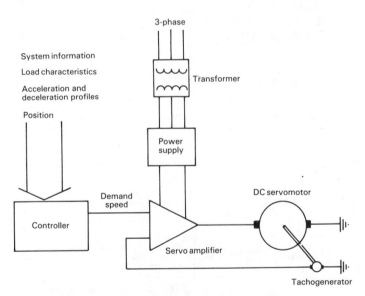

Fig. 4.13   Single axis drive configuration.

Typically, a DC servomotor uses a permanent magnet stator field with a wound armature and has the characteristics of a shunt motor. The servo amplifier, the full specification of which is given in Table 4.1, provides a full, four-quadrant pulse width modulated drive to the servomotor using a switching frequency of 3 kHz.

The servo amplifier circuit is shown in schematic form in Fig. 4.14. Control of the output pulse width is achieved by the controller integrated circuit. This receives the demand speed setting and compares this speed with the actual speed information supplied by the motor tachometer. From this comparison the controller then adjusts the firing of the Darlington drive transistors to balance the demand and actual speeds. The demand speed is set by an external control system which also

See Chapter 1 notes for the Darlington circuit.

Table 4.1 Renold Servo Amplifier Specification

Input		*Output*	
Power supply	75–90 V DC at 7.5 A continuous 20 A peak	Continous current	7.5 A
		Peak current	20 A for 5 s
Velocity	± 10 V DC	Deadband	Zero deadband
Tacho	12–20 V DC at maximum motor speed	Output waveform	PWM at 3 kHz
		Indicator lamps	Power on
			Forward enabled
Current limit	Adjustable from 10 to 20 A		Reverse enabled
			Over-temperature trip
Tacho gain	Adjustable between 12–10 V for maximum motor speed.		Over-current trip
			Over-voltage trip
			Current limit
Zero offset	Adjustable to ± 4% of velocity input	Fault relay	Volt-free contact rated at 240 V AC or 200 V DC at 0.5 A closes on operation of any of the three trips.
Forward enable	Enables forward rotation when connected to 0 V		
Reverse enable	Enables reverse rotation when connected to 0 V		
Drive enable	Enables forward and reverse rotation when connected to 0 V		

General			
Ambient temperature	0–40°C	Dust and moisture	IP 22

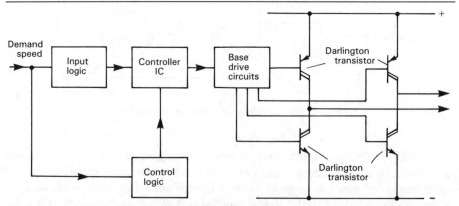

Fig. 4.14 Schematic of servo amplifier circuit. [Note: See Chapter 1, note 1.24 for the Darlington transistor.]

provides the necessary acceleration and deceleration profiles required for operation. A typical operating velocity/time profile produced by this external controller when used for positioning is shown by Fig. 4.15.

The servo amplifier also incorporates within itself the directional control logic,

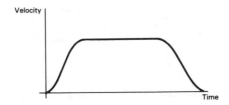

Fig. 4.15 Velocity-time profile for servo drive.

the condition of which will again be set by the external system, together with status and alarm logic. Trips include current and voltage limits as well as temperature. Status is shown by indicator lamps on the amplifier front panel.

(Incorporated with the permission of Renold plc)

A.C. Machines

Induction machines

In an induction machine a magnetic field rotating at synchronous speed is produced in the air gap by the polyphase stator winding. Provided the rotor is moving at a different speed to the field a voltage and hence a current will be induced into the short circuited rotor windings. The relationship between the rotor speed and the synchronous speed is expressed by the slip (s).

Synchronous speed in rpm = N_s
= 120 f/p
where f = supply frequency
and p = number of poles.
Synchronous speed in radians
$s^{-1} = \omega_s = 2\pi (N_s/60) = 2\pi f$
$\times 2/p = 2\omega/p$.

$$s = \frac{\text{Synchronous speed} - \text{Actual speed}}{\text{Synchronous speed}} \qquad (4.15)$$

Figure 4.16 shows the equivalent circuit for one phase of a polyphase induction machine. The internal mechanical power developed is

Ignores internal mechanical losses of machine such as windage and friction.

$$P_m = T_m\omega_m \qquad (4.16)$$
ω_m = Mechanical speed in radians s^{-1}

The power transferred across the airgap to the rotor is

$$P_{ag} = I_r'^2.R_r'/s \qquad (4.17)$$
Power loss in rotor resistance = $I_r'^2.R_r'$ \qquad (4.18)

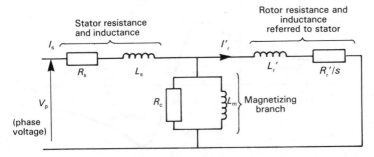

Fig. 4.16(a) Equivalent circuit of one phase of an induction machine.

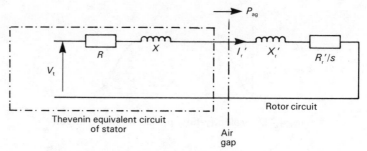

(b) Thevenin equivalent circuit of an induction motor

Fig. 4.16   Induction machine per phase equivalent circuits.

Energy converted to internal mechanical power =
$$I_r'^2.R_r'(1 - s)/s = P_{ag}(1 - s) \tag{4.19}$$

From Equation 4.15

$$\omega_m = (1 - s)\omega_s \tag{4.20}$$
ω_s = Synchronous speed in radians s^{-1}

Thus

$$T_m = P_{ag}/\omega_s = P_{ag} \, p/(2\omega)$$
$$= \frac{p}{2\omega} \left[\frac{V_t^2}{(R + R_r'/s)^2 + (X + X_r')^2} \right] \frac{R_r'}{s} \text{Nm/phase} \tag{4.21}$$

For an m phase machine

$$T_m = \frac{mp}{2\omega} \left[\frac{V_t^2}{(R + R_r'/s)^2 + (X + X_r')^2} \right] \frac{R_r'}{s} \text{Nm} \tag{4.22}$$

The curve of torque against speed (or slip) can now be obtained. A typical form, showing the various operating regions, is given as Fig. 4.17.

Braking

Electrical braking can be applied to an induction motor in a number of ways. If the direction of rotation of the magnetic field is reversed with respect to the direction of rotation of the rotor the slip is greater than unity and the machine operates in the

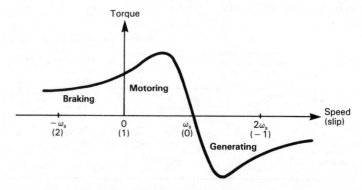

Fig. 4.17   Torque/speed characteristic of an induction machine.

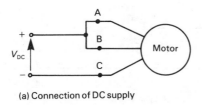

(a) Connection of DC supply

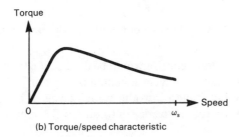

(b) Torque/speed characteristic

Fig. 4.18   D.C. dynamic braking of an induction motor.

braking region of Fig. 4.17. This is a very severe condition and will give rise to high currents in the machine windings. By reducing the supply frequency so that the field is rotating in the same direction as, but slower than, the rotor the slip becomes negative and the machine operates in the generating region, returning power to the supply.

ω_m is negative and slip is > 1.

$\omega_m > \omega_s$ and slip is negative.

For DC dynamic braking the AC supply is disconnected and a DC supply connected as in Fig. 4.18(a). This produces a stationary magnetic field and gives the braking characteristic of Fig. 4.18(b).

Voltage control

If the voltage applied to an induction machine is varied at fixed frequency the torque/speed characteristic will vary as shown by Fig. 4.19. This will enable a limited degree of speed variation to be obtained but at a decrease in efficiency with decreasing speed, since

$$\text{Efficiency} \simeq (1 - s) \qquad (4.23)$$

A simple means of achieving this form of control is to use a reverse parallel pair of thyristors in each phase of the supply as in Fig. 4.20.

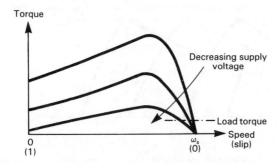

Fig. 4.19   Torque/speed characteristic with voltage control.

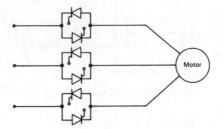

Fig. 4.20   Voltage control of an induction motor.

Speed variation by voltage control would be used over a limited speed range only and at a restricted torque to prevent machine overheating. This form of control also has the disadvantage that it introduces high levels of harmonic currents into the supply system as a result of the discontinuity of the supply current waveform.

Variable-frequency operation

The maximum torque produced by an induction motor is given by

$$T_{max} = \frac{mp}{4\omega} \; \frac{V_t^2}{R + [R^2 + (X + X_r')^2]^{1/2}} \tag{4.24}$$

Ignoring R, Equation 4.24 may be approximated by

$$T_{max} = \frac{mp}{4\omega} \; \frac{V_t^2}{(X + X_r')} = \frac{mp}{4(L + L_r')} \; \frac{V_t^2}{\omega^2} \tag{4.25}$$

Therefore, to maintain T_{max} constant

$$V_p/f = \text{constant} \tag{4.26}$$

which results in the torque/speed relationship of Fig. 4.21. In practice, the voltage would be increased above the nominal value of Equation 4.26 at low speeds to overcome the effects of the stator resistance.

These conditions can be met by the circuit of Fig. 4.22. The voltage-sourced inverter may be of the squarewave or quasi-squarewave type when the voltage is controlled by variation of the DC level, either by control of the AC input via a controlled converter or a diode bridge supplying a DC chopper. Where the DC link

See Chapter 3 for operation of a voltage sourced inverter.

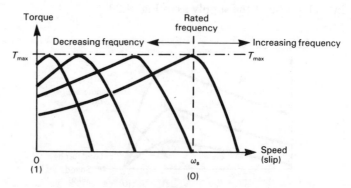

Fig. 4.21   Ideal torque/speed characteristic of an induction machine with V/f constant.

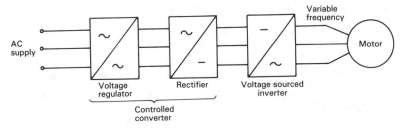

Fig. 4.22   Induction motor with voltage sourced inverter.

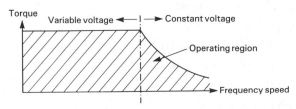

Compare with Fig. 4.6 for a DC machine.

Fig. 4.23   Operating envelope of an induction motor with variable frequency control.

voltage is used directly for the commutation capacitors the commutation requirements will determine the minimum DC voltage that can be used. To overcome this limitation a commutation system which uses a higher voltage derived directly from the supply could be adopted. Operation of an inverter with variable output voltage for induction motor control is limited usually to frequencies above about 5 Hz to prevent drive instabilities occurring.

The diode bridge could also be used in conjunction with a pulse-width-modulated inverter for operation up to the maximum voltage condition. If operation is required beyond this point then the inverter would be arranged to provide a squarewave or quasi-squarewave supply to the motor at a constant voltage. This results in the torque/speed envelope of Fig. 4.23.

Normally, the chopping frequency (f_c) used by the pulse-width-modulated inverter would be an exact multiple of the inverter output frequency (f_i), with the ratio f_c/f_i changed at regular speed intervals. At low frequencies, f_c is usually kept constant to avoid excess current ripple, the loss of synchronization with f_i being taken account of by the large number of pulses in each half cycle which reduces the variation between cycles.

The ratio f_c/f_i is varied normally in steps from around 150:1 at low frequencies to 15:1 for f_i above 50 Hz. The process of changing this ratio is referred to as 'gear changing'.

Worked Example 4.3

The equivalent circuit for a four-pole, three-phase induction machine operating at 50 Hz is shown in the figure. What will be the maximum torque produced under the following conditions?

(i) 240 V/phase,   50 Hz;   (ii) 120 V/phase,   50 Hz;   (iii) 60 V/phase;   50 Hz; (iv) 96 V/phase, 20 Hz;   (v) 24 V/phase, 5 Hz.

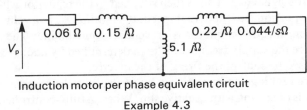

Induction motor per phase equivalent circuit

Example 4.3

Thevenin equivalent circuit parameters at 50 Hz

$$|V_t| = \left| \frac{5.1j \times V}{0.06 + 0.152j + 5.1j} \right| = 0.9711 \times V$$

$$Z_t = \frac{5.1j\,(0.06 + 0.152j)}{0.06 + 0.152; + 5.1j} = 0.158\,|69.12° = 0.0563 + 0.148j\ \Omega$$

From Equation 4.24

$$T_{max} = \frac{3 \times 4}{4 \times 2 \times 50 \times \pi} \times \frac{V_t^2}{0.0563 + [0.0563^2 + (0.148 + 0.22)^2]^{1/2}}$$
$$= 0.02229 \times V_t^2 \text{ at 50 Hz}$$

(i) $V_t = 0.9711 \times 240 = 233$ V
     $T_{max} = 0.02229 \times 233^2 = 1210$ Nm

(ii) $V_t = 0.9711 \times 120 = 116.5$ V
     $T_{max} = 0.02229 \times 116.5^2 = 302.7$ Nm

(iii) $V_t = 0.9711 \times 60 = 58.3$ V
     $T_{max} = 0.02229 \times 58.3^2 = 75.7$ Nm

(iv) $|V_t| = \left| \dfrac{\frac{2}{5} \times 5.1j \times 96}{0.06 + \frac{2}{5}(0.152 + 5.1)j} \right| = 93.17$ V

$$Z_t = \frac{\frac{2}{5} \times 5.1j\,(0.06 + \frac{2}{5} \times 0.152j)}{0.06 + \frac{2}{5}\,(0.152 + 5.1)j} = 0.0565 + 0.0606j\ \Omega$$

$$T_{max} = \frac{3 \times 4}{4 \times 2 \times 20 \times \pi} \times \frac{93.17^2}{0.0565 + [0.0565^2 + (0.0606 + \frac{2}{5} \times 0.22)^2]^{1/2}}$$
$$= 962 \text{ Nm}$$

(v) $V_t = \left| \dfrac{\frac{1}{10} \times 5.1j \times 24}{0.06\,\frac{1}{10}\,(0.152 + 5.1)j} \right| = 23.16$ V

$$Z_t = \frac{\frac{1}{10} \times 5.1j\,(0.06 + \frac{1}{10} \times 0.152j)}{0.06 + \frac{1}{10}\,(0.152 + 5.1)j} = 0.0558 + 0.0212j\ \Omega$$

$$T_{max} = \frac{3 \times 4}{4 \times 2 \times 5 \times \pi} \cdot \frac{23.16^2}{0.0558 + [0.0558^2 + (0.0212 + \frac{1}{10} \times 0.22)^2]^{1/2}}$$
$$= 405.3 \text{ Nm}$$

The effect of the winding resistance in reducing the maximum torque from the ideal value at lower frequencies is seen clearly from results (i), (iv) and (v).

Figure 4.24 shows a typical speed controller for a constant-speed inverter drive. The demand speed (ω_r) is compared with the signal from the tachogenerator (ω_a) to produce an error signal (ω_e). This is then supplied to the regulator which sets a slip speed (ω_{slip}) proportional to the actual speed. By limiting ω_{slip} to a value corresponding to maximum torque the motor is prevented from stalling. The synchronous speed and hence the supply frequency is then determined by adding ω_s and ω_a and this signal is used to control the firing of the inverter.

Regenerative braking can be achieved by controlling the inverter frequency so that the motor is operating with negative slip. Where a fully-controlled converter is

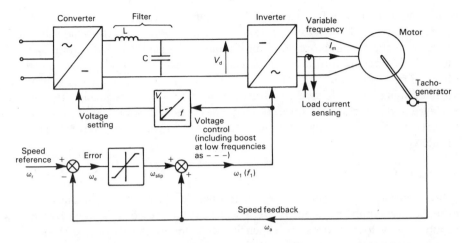

Fig. 4.24   Control system for induction motor with voltage sourced inverter.

used to obtain the DC supply for the inverter the regenerative power can be fed back into the main AC supply. If a half-controlled converter is used then a braking resistor can be connected in the DC link at the input to the inverter to absorb the regenerated power. In this latter case additional control must be provided to prevent the voltage of the DC link rising to too high a value. One method of achieving this control is by switching a transistor in series with the braking resistor.

Braking circuit.

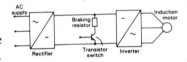

Current-sourced inverter

A current-sourced inverter is used where rapid changes of output torque are to be avoided as the inductance of the DC link prevents rapid changes of motor current. The control systems for a current-sourced inverter drive tend to be more complex than those for a voltage-sourced inverter drive. Figure 4.25 shows a typical

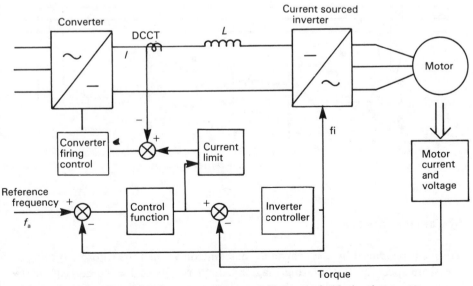

Fig. 4.25   Controller for a current sourced inverter fed induction motor.

101

controller. The inverter frequency (f_i) is compared with the demand frequency (f_d) and the error signal taken as input to the controller which sets the magnitude and direction of the demand torque, ensuring that this is kept within the limits for the motor. This demand torque is compared with an assessment of the actual torque obtained from measured values of motor voltage, current and frequency to provide an error signal which is used to adjust the inverter output frequency. Braking is achieved by reducing the inverter frequency when the inverter input voltage reverses, putting the supply converter into the inverting mode and returning power to the AC supply.

Cycloconverter drives

Where operation is required only at frequencies below the frequency of the available AC supply, a cycloconverter may be used to provide a variable-frequency supply. As cycloconverters are expensive in terms of the number of switching devices used and the complexity of their control systems, their application tends to be limited to situations where high powers are required at the lower end of the speed range.

Slip-ring induction machine

It is possible with an induction machine having a wound rotor to bring the ends of the rotor windings to slip rings, allowing access to the rotor circuit. This has led to the development of the slip energy recovery controllers in which energy is extracted from the rotor at rotor frequency and returned via a frequency converter to the supply. By controlling the amount of recovered energy the speed of the machine can be controlled. One version of this type of controller is the static Kramer drive of Fig. 4.26 in which the frequency conversion is performed by a rectifier and converter combination.

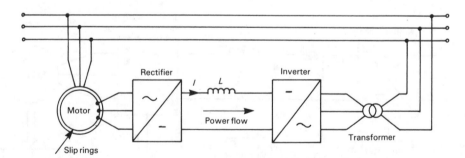

Fig. 4.26   Static Kramer system.

Synchronous machine

Torque is produced by a synchronous machine only when the rotor is rotating at the same speed as the rotating magnetic field produced by the current in the polyphase stator winding. The simple per-phase equivalent circuit for a

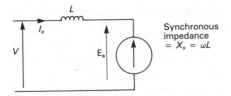

Fig. 4.27 Per phase equivalent circuit of a synchronous machine.

synchronous machine is shown in Fig. 4.27. From this figure the per-phase power is

$$\text{Power} = VI_a \cos \phi = VE_a \sin \delta / X \qquad (4.27)$$

where δ is the load angle and defines the angle between the stator and rotor fields in the airgap of the machine. As the synchronous machine operates at a fixed speed determined by the frequency of the supply to the stator up to its maximum load, it can be fed from any of the forms of inverter already described.

For a 3-phase machine total power $= 3VI_a \cos \phi$
$= V_{line}E_{a,line} \sin \delta / X$.

The speed at which the synchronous machine operates is synchronous speed and has the same value as the synchronous speed of an induction motor with the same number of poles.

Brushless machines

In the brushless machine the field circuit is replaced by a powerful permanent magnet, eliminating the need for a commutator and brushgear. Construction is typically as in Fig. 4.28 with the permanent magnets mounted on the rotor and a stator winding connected as shown. The advantages of the resulting machine are reduced maintainance, increased torque/volume ratio, availability of peak torque to high speed and simplified protection. As a result, machines of this type have found increasing application as servo motors in robots and machine tools.

Samarium Cobalt or other rare earth magnets are used to obtain the required flux densities.

The brushless machine can be operated either as a synchronous machine, in which case it would receive a variable-frequency, multi-phase supply, or as a DC machine with the commutation performed electrically. Of the two options the synchronous machine mode has the more complex control system by virtue of the need to control the inverter to produce the multi-phase, variable-frequency supply. Operation is, however, likely to be more flexible than as a DC machine.

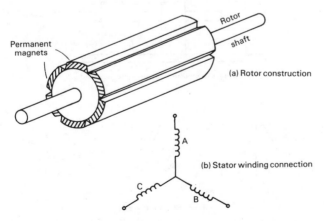

(a) Rotor construction

(b) Stator winding connection

Fig. 4.28 Brushless motor construction and connection.

180° (electrical) = 180°
(mechanical) × 2/(Number of
poles).

See also the switched
reluctance motor.

When operated as a DC machine the DC source is connected between the pairs of terminals of Fig. 4.28(b) in the sequence AB-AC-BC-BA-CA-CB-AB, switching taking place every 60° (electrical). The actual point at which commutation takes place is determined by reference to the rotor position, either by monitoring the shaft position or by using Hall Effect devices to sense the magnetic field.

The brushless motor can exhibit a ripple in its output torque. The major components of this ripple are the reluctance ripple caused by the inherent magnetic asymmetry of the machine and a drive current ripple at a frequency of $pn/2$, where p is the number of poles and n is the speed in r/min. There is also a component, known as the once-round ripple, at a frequency corresponding to the rotational speed of the machine, which is caused by the non-alignment of the rotor within the stator. Ripple can be reduced by control of the supply to the motor, aided by the use of a microprocessor-based controller to optimize switching performance.

Stepper Motors

Variable reluctance

Figure 4.29(a) shows a three-stack, variable-reluctance stepper motor with each stack having four poles. When the poles of stack I are energized the rotor aligns itself with these poles as in Fig. 4.29(b). If these poles are then de-energized and the poles of stack II are energized, the rotor moves one step in a clockwise direction. By varying the number of stacks, the number of poles per stack and the number of teeth per pole, the size of the step can be controlled such that

Step angle = $360/(sn)$

where s = number of stacks
n = number of teeth per stack = number of poles × teeth per pole.

The windings from each stack are referred to as a phase and can be connected in any of the ways of Fig. 4.30.

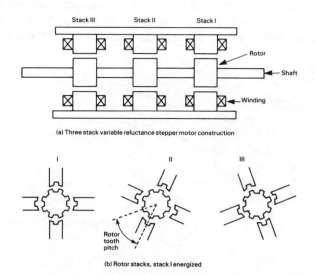

(a) Three stack variable reluctance stepper motor construction

(b) Rotor stacks, stack I energized

Fig. 4.29   Four pole, three stack variable reluctance stepper motor.

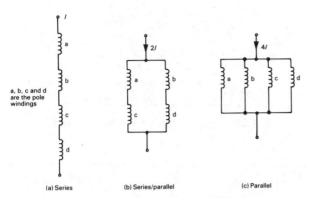

Fig. 4.30   Connection of pole windings on one stack (phase) of a four pole, variable reluctance stepper motor.

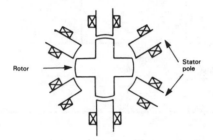

Fig. 4.31   Single stack, variable reluctance stepper motor configuration.

As an alternative to the multi-stack design the configuration of Fig. 4.31 can be used in which the rotor and stator have different pole numbers. By energizing the stator phases in sequence the rotor can be stepped as before, with half steps or other incremental steps achieved by energizing two phases together. The step angle is given by

Step angle = $360/(Mn)$

where M = number of phases
n = number of rotor teeth.

Hybrid

The hybrid stepper motor, shown in Fig. 4.32, has a permanent magnet on the rotor together with two windings on the stator which excite alternate poles. By energizing the windings positively and negatively in sequence the rotor can be stepped in either direction. A complete switching cycle consists of four steps, after which the excitation state is back to its initial form. The step angle is therefore.

Step angle = $90/n$

where n = is the number of teeth on the rotor.

The hybrid motor generally operates with a smaller step angle than the variable-reluctance motor and has a higher torque/volume ratio. It can also provide a holding or detent torque when the stator is unexcited.

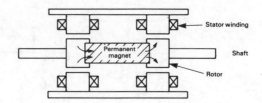

Fig. 4.32 Hybrid stepper motor construction.

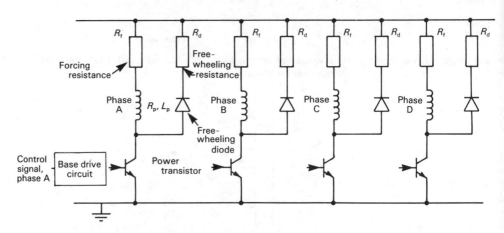

Fig. 4.33 Drive circuit for a four phase, variable reluctance stepper motor.

Drive circuits

The variable-reluctance stepper has at least four phases which can be supplied from a DC source as the direction of current in the windings for operation is unimportant. The hybrid motor on the other hand requires a drive circuit which will reverse the direction of current in the two phases. The simplest drive for the variable-reluctance stepper is that shown in Fig. 4.33. As the phase winding has significant inductance the forcing resistance R_f is included to reduce the time constant and allow operation over a wider speed range. On turn-off the energy stored in the inductance of the phase winding is dissipated via the freewheeling diode across the winding. The voltage across the transistor on turn-off is

$$V_{CE} = V_s + IR_d \tag{4.28}$$

Where a bi-directional current is required the circuit of Fig. 4.34 is used. By switching the transistors in pairs the required current direction is achieved.

Switched reluctance motor

One form of the switched reluctance motor is shown in Fig. 4.35. Simultaneously exciting a diametrically opposite pair of poles causes a pair of rotor poles to be attracted magnetically into alignment with the excited poles, providing the basic torque mechanism. If a subsequent pair of poles (BB') in sequence were then excited a further rotation would take place.

The transistors must be chosen and rated to handle the highest switching frequency. See Chapter 1.

Time constant = L/R. Requires V_s to be increased.

Compare with the stepper motor.

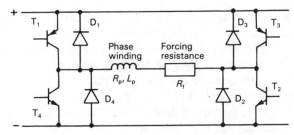

Fig. 4.34 Bi-directional current drive circuit. [Compare with Fig. 3.13 for the voltage sourced; single phase inverter.]

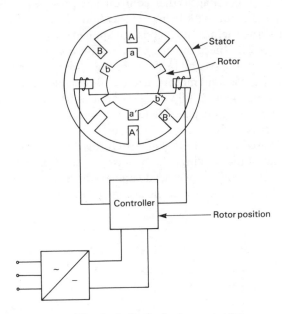

Fig. 4.35 Switched reluctance motor.

If the stator is supplied with a constant voltage and switching takes place at a fixed rotor position relative to the stator poles, the machine would provide a DC series motor torque/speed characteristic. By varying the rotor position at which switching takes place in combination with control of the current, a range of operating characteristics is made available.

Operation therefore requires that the controller makes reference to the rotor position in order to establish the pattern of switching the stator winding and hence some form of positional feedback must be provided.

Traction Drives

Traction drives have traditionally used the DC series motor with its high torque at low speeds. Early designs using on-board rectifiers and tap-changing transformers operated with up to 30% ripple in the motor supply, smoothed by the machine inductance and added series inductance. The advent of power electronics has increased the flexibility of operation by allowing the machine designer to optimize

Limit on the permitted ripple is set by the effect on communications and signalling circuits.

107

performance over the full operating envelope of the machine and has led to the introduction of drives using separately excited DC motors and AC motors. The incorporation of microprocessor-based controllers has optimized tractive effort by allowing operation close to the limit of adhesion, has enabled greater use to be made of regenerative braking and has permitted the development of new traction technologies such as linear motors.

Figure 4.36 shows a simplified locomotive traction system using multiple converters and operating from an AC supply. Reversal is achieved by reverse-parallel converters supplying the field windings.

The normal AC supply voltage for a traction system is single phase at 25 kV.

On start-up from rest, full field is applied to the motors and one bridge in each group is fired. Its output voltage is then controlled to provide a constant current to the motors, the conduction path being via the diode arms of the inactive bridge. The vehicle will then accelerate under constant applied torque. As the back EMF of the motors increases with speed the firing angle of the conducting bridge is brought to zero, at which point the second bridge is brought into full operation. Acceleration then continues at constant motor current and constant torque until the second bridge is fully conducting and full voltage is applied to the traction motors. Any further speed control is by means of field variation.

Field weakening.

Where the power is derived from a DC source then a chopper drive would be used. This can be based on any of the standard forms described and could use either regenerative or rheostatic braking. For a railway system the DC source could be picked up from a third rail or overhead catenary or generated on-board as on a diesel electric locomotive. For road vehicles the power source would be on-board batteries.

Standard DC voltages are 600 V, 750 V, 1500 V and 3000 V.

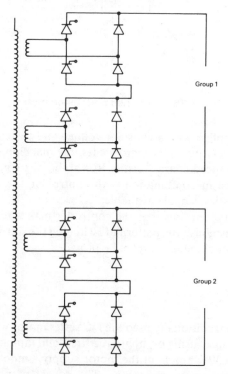

Fig. 4.36 Converter arrangement for a locomotive traction drive with separate control of the motors on each bogie.

Developments in traction systems include the use of inverters to supply both conventional and linear induction motors, the application of the switched-reluctance motors and the development of new controllers and control strategies based on the application of microprocessor technologies.

Worked Example 4.4

For a traction system of the type shown in Fig. 4.36, the rectifiers are each supplied with 320 V at 50 Hz from the 25 kV, 50 Hz supply. If the motor voltage in each group is three-quarters of its maximum value and the total motor current in each group is constant at 1200 A, estimate the RMS value of the current drawn from the 25 kV supply. Neglect all losses.

For three-quarters maximum voltage at the motors one bridge is fully conducting ($\alpha = 0°$) and the other is providing half its maximum output voltage ($\alpha = 90°$).

Transformer ratio = 25000/320 = 78.125

Current in primary due to the fully conducting bridges is

$$I_{p1} = 2 \times 320 \times 1200/25000 = 30.72 \text{ A continuous.}$$

Current in primary due to the bridge operating at half maximum output voltage is

$$I_{p2} = 2 \times 320 \times 1200/2500 = 30.72 \text{ A for 50\% of the time.}$$

The RMS current in the 25 kV system is therefore

$$I_{25kV} = \left[\frac{1}{2\pi} \left(\int_0^\pi 30.72^2 \, d\theta + \int_0^\pi 61.44^2 \, d\theta \right) \right]^{½}$$
$$= 48.57 \text{ A}$$

Case Study — The BR Maglev System, GEC Transportation Projects

The British Rail Maglev system has its origins in work carried out in the 1970s at the British Rail Technical Centre in Derby based upon developments in magnet and control technologies since the 1950s. The approach adopted was to suspend the vehicle by means of an upward attractive force produced by electromagnets on a steel track, with a linear induction motor to provide the propulsive force. Though this means of suspension is inherently unstable it proved possible to control the system electronically to maintain a mean gap of 15 mm.

On the basis of this development work the BR Maglev system was chosen for the passenger link between Birmingham International Airport and the National Exhibition Centre (NEC) in competition with other, more conventional, forms of transport. The system, details of which are given in Table 4.2, is intended to provide a shuttle service with a design capacity of 2215 passengers per hour over a track length of 623 metres. Two-car trains each with a maximum payload of three tonnes run on parallel tracks with a maximum speed of 42 km/h. The whole of the system can be operated from a single control desk. Provision is made for features such as unmanned operation, programmed service frequency or passenger call

Table 4.2   Birmingham International Airport/NEC Maglev System Details

System Design		*System Performance*	
Configuration	Dual independent tracks on an elevated guideway. Stations at each end, substation in middle.	Acceleration	1.24 m/s² max.
		Emergency braking rate	2 m/s²
		Clamp-up deceleration	5 m/s²
		Jerk	1.25 m/s³ max.
Track length	623 m buffer-to-buffer	Speed	15 m/s = 54 km/h = 34 mile/h
Passenger flow	190 per direction per 15 min	Vertical ride	0.045 g
Track capacity	397 passengers per 15 min or 274 passengers + luggage per direction per 15 min	Lateral ride	0.033 g (0.08 g on curve)
		Longitudinal ride	0.033 g
		Lateral natural frequency	1.5 Hz
Car capacity	34 standing, 6 seated	Stopping accuracy	±100 mm
		Max roll angle	±2.6°
Frequency	8 train trips/ 15 min	Max pitch angle	±1.26°
		Max yaw angle	±1.3°
Journey time	100 s	Emergency braking distance	50 m max. (ice-free)
Dwell time	44 s nominal. Adjustable 5 to 90s.	Energy consumption	2 kWh per vehicle journey
Floor space	98 m² per direction per 15 min		
Noise level	60 to 66 dBA 3 m from track at 13 m/s, 75 dBA inside vehicle.		

Track requirements			
Design life	50 years	Max gradient	1.5%
Banking	None	Curve, horizontal, min.	40 m radius
Level	±5 mm, −10 mm abs.		
Rate of change	1 in 500 on 10 mm chord	Curve, vertical, min.	1400 m radius
		Alignment	±4 mn, −4 mm, 10 mm chord

Vehicle	
Length	6.00 m external; 5.54 m internal
Width	2.25 m external; 1.85 m internal
Height	3.50 m external; 2.23 m internal
Weights	5000 kg empty; 8000 kg loaded (3000 kg payload)

service. Safety systems are designed on a fail-to-safe basis with appropriate back-up systems.

The project was carried out by a consortium of British companies with GEC Transportation Projects as the project managers. Construction began in 1981 and the system entered partial public service on 7 August 1984 and full service soon thereafter.

The consortium operated under the name of 'People Mover Group'.

The track

The track system adopted is shown in Fig. 4.37 and is carried on a concrete structure five metres above ground. Alignment incorporates two curves of about fifty metres radius and a gradient of 1.5%. A removable track section is included for vehicle removal. The track itself is constructed of steel sleepers carrying the laminated steel support rails, a pair of aluminium power supply rails at 600 V and the reaction rail for the linear induction motor. Also included in the track system are cable loops for communication between the vehicle and trackside and marker plates for overspeed detection. Docking at the stations is to within ± 100 mm with a maximum gap between the platform and vehicle of 55 mm.

Power supply

The track power supply of 600 V, 700 A, DC is fed from the incoming 11 kV AC system by transformer/rectifiers, with separate supplies for each track. To prevent stray currents and associated interference and corrosion problems, single-point

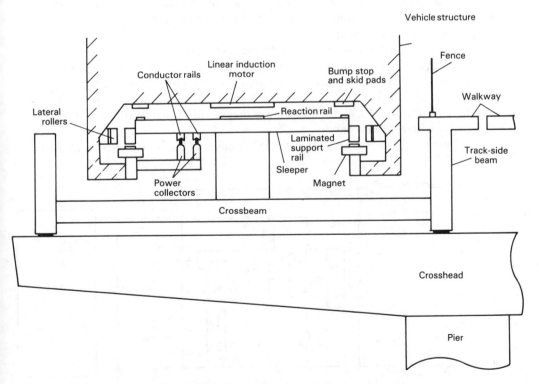

Fig. 4.37 Maglev track system.

earthing at the substation is used. The vehicle collects power via metallized carbon collector shoes running in channels on the conductor rails.

On board the vehicles, auxiliaries are supplied from a 3 kW, 600/48 V DC/DC converter with a 24 Ah lead–acid battery backup. Load shedding is used on a failure of the main supply, allowing sensitive loads to be maintained for about twenty minutes.

Control and communications

Control and communication is based upon the following systems:

(a) The Automatic Train Protection (ATP) system dealing with safety functions.
(b) The Automatic Train Operation (ATO) system performing the driving functions.
(c) The supervision system interfacing with the control-room operator.
(d) The communications system providing a link between the operator and the passengers.

Operation can either be continuous with running on one or both tracks with a preset dwell time at each station or on-demand when the vehicles run on response to passenger requests. Starting is under control of the central or local scheduling logic with running operation controlled by the ATO computer.

Suspension and Guidance

A magnetic suspension system must control the inherently unstable suspension gap in relation to ride quality, taking into account factors such as the interaction between the suspension control and the resonances of both the supporting structure and the vehicle.

The suspension system uses eight magnets mounted in pairs at the vehicle corners, the magnets of each pair being laterally offset on opposite sides of the rail centre line to provide guidance. The magnets operate with a nominal gap of 15 mm and an airgap flux density of 0.8 tesla. The average power for levitation and control is about 3 kW/tonne giving a magnet lift/weight ratio of the order of 11.7:1 with a 15 mm gap.

The magnet pairs are driven by the DC chopper of Fig. 4.38, together for vertical

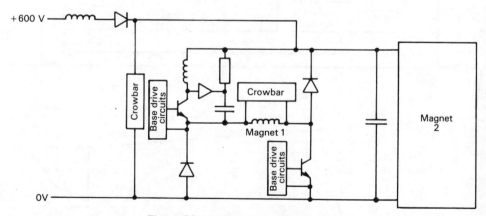

Fig. 4.38 Levitation power system.

control and guidance and differentially for lateral damping. Each of the two-quadrant bridge circuits is switching in anti-phase at 1 kHz. Chopper efficiency is 97%. On turn-on the base current is held at about 2 A for about 6 μs before falling to a lower value. There is also a high initial collector current pulse due to the discharge of the snubber capacitor. During turn-off an LC circuit is used to provide a high peak reverse current in the base circuit to optimize turn-off performance. A complete turn-on or turn-off takes about 8 μs.

See Chapter 1 for conditions for rapid turn-on and turn-off of transistors.

Protection of the power transistors is included within the base drive circuit while separate crowbar thyristors are used to protect both the power supply and the levitation magnets.

Stability of the suspension system is obtained by ensuring that the magnet currents can be adjusted more rapidly than changes of magnetic force produced by the magnets can occur. Vertical damping is obtained by using a signal proportional to the rate of change of the air gap. The restoring forces introduced by offsetting the magnet pairs means that the guidance system is inherently stable but requires some lateral damping. This is achieved by differentially exciting each pair of magnets to ensure the resulting vertical force is constant. The additional lateral force ensures stability.

Propulsion and braking

The propulsion system is shown in Fig. 4.39 and uses an inverter-driven, short-stator, single-sided, axial-flux linear induction motor mounted centrally under the vehicle. The reaction rail is a steel beam capped by an aluminium plate and fixed to the suspension rail. The motor develops a tractive thrust of 4 kN from rest to 15 m/s with a maximum continuous rating of 2 kN at 15 m/s at an operational air gap for the motor of 20 mm.

The inverter is of the pulse-width-modulated type using transistor switching

The linear induction motor system was supplied by Brush Electrical Mechines Ltd.

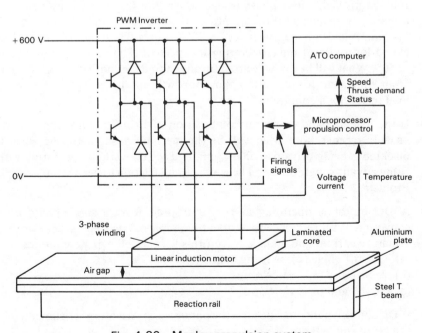

Fig. 4.39   Maglev propulsion system.

modules and is rated at 240 kVA continuously or 325 kVA (450 A) for 60 s. The output frequency range is 0 to 45 Hz at power factors in the range 0.5 to 0.9, lagging or leading.

Waveform generation, inverter control and protection are achieved by means of a microprocessor-based controller. The inverter control will respond to a demand by the ATO computer, taking into account vehicle speed, line voltage, motor current, motor airgap and jerk limit. The slip is adjusted to give either a motoring or a braking force. The velocity profile is matched to the track alignment and the required acceleration and deceleration rates.

Cooling of the motor is achieved by air ducted over the core and winding with a blower automatically cutting-in if the winding exceeds a specified temperature. The inverter uses natural air cooling via fins on the exterior of the vehicle.

(Based on: Nenadovic, V. and Riches, E.E. (1985). Maglev at Birmingham Airport: from system concept to successful operation. *GEC Review* **1** (1). Reproduced with permission of GEC).

> Jerk is the rate of acceleration (d^2 (velocity)/dt^2 = ms^{-3}). The jerk limit applied for the Maglev system is 0.6 ms^{-3}.

Problems

4.1 Referring to Worked Example 4.2, the DC motor is operating from a 240 V (RMS) supply and is developing a mean torque of 2 Nm. The thyristors are being fired at $\alpha = 100°$ and the armature current continues for 45° beyond the voltage zero. If the motor has a torque constant ($K\phi$) of 1 Nm/A and an armature resistance of 4.8 Ω, what will be the motor speed under these conditions? Neglect all mechanical losses in the motor.

4.2 A separately excited DC motor is supplied from a 415 V, 50 Hz supply by a fully-controlled, single phase bridge converter. The motor parameters are: armature resistance 5.4 Ω, armature inductance 48 mH, torque constant 1.4 Nm/A and voltage constant ($K\phi$) 1.4 V/rad/s. The motor is operated with closed-loop control and is operating at a speed of 1800 rpm with a firing angle of 50°. What will be the net output torque? Windage and friction are constant at an equivalent torque of 0.6 Nm. How will the firing angle vary from no load to full load conditions?

4.3 If the machine and converter combination of Problem 2 are configured to provide regeneration, what will be the mechanical input torque when the machine is being driven at 2000 r/min and the converter is operating with a firing advance angle of 36°? The windage and friction losses are the same as in Problem 2.

4.4 A DC motor is operating at constant speed from a single-phase bridge converter. With reference to Worked Example 4.2 and Fig. 2.26, sketch the armature current and voltage waveforms for the following conditions:
   (a) Cut-off angle (ψ) > firing angle (α) > ($\sigma - \pi$)
   (b) $\psi > \alpha$ and ($\sigma - \pi$) > α
   (c) $\psi > \alpha$ and ($\sigma - \pi$) = ψ

4.5 A DC shunt-wound machine has the parameters: Armature resistance 0.78 Ω, armature inductance 16 mH, torque constant 2.1 Nm/A and voltage constant 0.209 V/r/min. It is supplied by a fully controlled, three-phase bridge converter from a 220 V (line), 50 Hz AC source. Find expressions for the armature current and hence determine the values for mean torque, speed, etc, as appropriate for the following conditions:

(a) Motoring with a firing angle of 22.5°, a continuous current and 70 Nm torque.
(b) Generating with a firing advance angle of 22.5°, a continuous current and 70 Nm torque.
(c) Motoring with a firing angle of 67.5° at a speed of 720 r/min.
(d) Generating at a firing advance angle of 67.5° at a speed of 720 r/min.

4.6 For the three-phase induction machine of Worked Example 4.3, find the values of supply voltage required to maintain the maximum torque constant for each of the operating conditions given in the example.

4.7 A static Kramer system is used to control an eight-pole, slip ring induction machine from a 415 V (line), 50 Hz supply, with the inverter connected directly to the supply. Find the firing advance angle of the inverter when the motor is operating at 660 rpm. The rectifier operates with an overlap angle of 18° and the inverter with an overlap angle of 4.2°. The diodes and thyristors have forward voltage drops of 1.1 and 1.6 V respectively. The open-circuit voltage measured at the slip rings with the machine stationary is 720 V.
(Note: When motoring, Slip-ring voltage = (Open-circuit slip-ring voltage) × slip.)

.5 Applications II

Objectives

☐ To examine the application of power semiconductors to high-voltage DC transmission.

☐ To consider voltage regulation circuits.

☐ To consider a range of power supplies, including switched-mode and series-resonant power supplies.

☐ To consider the operation of the thyristor circuit-breaker.

☐ To examine briefly the influence of microprocessor and microelectronics technologies on power electronics.

High-voltage DC Transmission

Kimbark, E.W. (1971). *Direct Current Transmission: Volume 1*. John Wiley, New York.

AC transmission dominates electricity supply by virtue of ease of generation, motor characteristics and the ability to change voltage magnitudes using transformers. High-voltage DC (HVDC) transmission uses a lighter and cheaper construction, with one or two conductors instead of three, but requires complex and expensive terminal arrangements. However, where power is to be transmitted over long distances, either overhead or with cables, or when a connection is required between systems operating at different frequencies, HVDC may well become economic. This has led to the installation worldwide of a number of HVDC links operating at powers of several gigawatts with voltages of ± 500 V DC or higher. Figure 5.1 illustrates the growth of HVDC transmission to 1983 when

The first modern HVDC scheme was the 96 km Gotland Link installed in 1954 between Vostervik in Sweden and Visby in Gotland. This was a monopolar link with sea return operating in 100 kV and 20 MW.

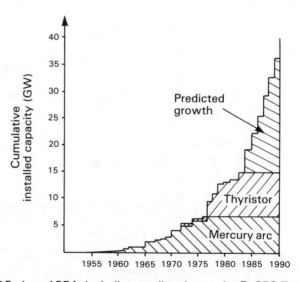

Fig. 5.1   HVDC since 1954, including predicted growth. © GEC Transmission and Distribution Projects.

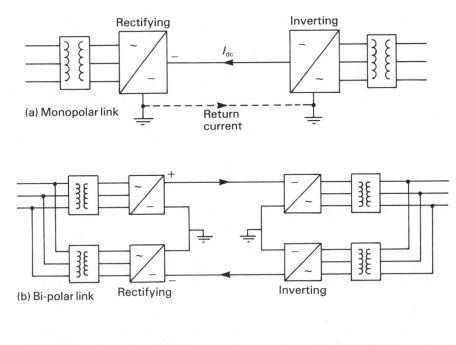

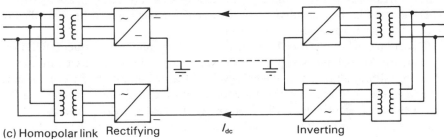

(c) Homopolar link   Rectifying I_{dc} Inverting

Fig. 5.2   Types of HVDC link.

there was an approximately equal division between systems using solid-state devices (thyristors) and mercury-arc valves. The shape of the curve from 1984 on indicates the predicted growth in HVDC to 1990.

Figure 5.2 shows the basic types of HVDC transmission system. The simplest arrangement is the monopolar link of Fig. 5.2(a) which uses a single conductor, usually at negative polarity, with a ground or sea return. The bipolar link of Fig. 5.2(b) has both a positive and a negative conductor and each terminal consists of a pair of converters connected in series on the DC side and in parallel on the AC side. The neutral points are grounded at one or both ends. With both ends grounded the poles can operate independently. Normally, operation is with equal current in the positive and negative conductors as there is then no earth current. In the case of a fault on one conductor the other can supply half the rated load using the earth return. A homopolar link has a number of conductors at the same polarity, normally negative, and earth return.

An HVDC converter will consist typically of a pair of six-pulse bridges connected in parallel on the AC side and in series on the DC side as in Fig. 5.3. By introducing a phase shift of 30° between the outputs of the supply transformers

Negative polarity is preferred as it produces less radio interference.

117

Each of the thyristors in
Fig. 5.3 is in fact a 'thyristor
valve' group.

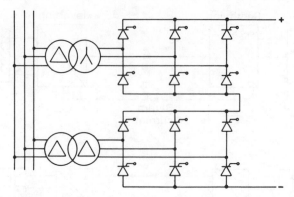

Fig. 5.3   HVDC twelve pulse converter formed by the connection of two six pulse
converters.

The term 'thyristor valve' is
used in HVDC systems to refer
to the connection of a number
of thyristors in series/parallel to
provide the required current and
voltage ratings. See Chapter 1
for discussion of the connection
of thyristors in series and
parallel.

this connection results in an effective twelve-pulse operation. In practice, each of the *'thyristor valves'* shown is made up of a number of individual devices connected in series/parallel to provide the necessary current and voltage ratings.

Typical control schemes include constant DC current and constant DC voltage, equidistant firing angle operation and, in the case of the inverting station, operation with a constant extinction angle. Protection would also be incorporated in the control scheme. For example, in the case of a fault resulting in an increase in the DC current in the transmission system the firing angle would be controlled to prevent the current exceeding a preset limit.

DC current can be measured by means of the DC current transformer (DCCT) of Fig. 5.4. An AC voltage is applied to the secondary coils which are connected in series opposition. During any one half cycle of the AC supply the flux in one core will add to the DC flux, causing that core to saturate, and subtract from the DC flux in the other core. There will then be no induced voltage in the coil of the saturated core since $d\phi/dt$ is zero during saturation while an ampere-turns balance will be set up in the coil of the unsaturated core. The AC source current will assume a value such that:

$$\text{AC source current} = \text{DC load current} \times \text{turns ratio} \qquad (5.1)$$

to maintain the core in the unsaturated state and balancing the AC voltage. This means that the output current of the rectifier is related to the DC system current by the turns ratio of the DCCT. More recently, measuring devices based on the Hall Effect have come into use for measuring DC current levels.

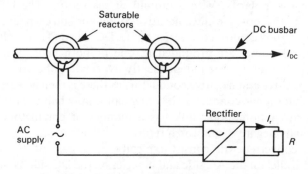

Fig. 5.4   D.C. current transformer (DCCT).

Case Study — Cross-Channel Link
(GEC Transmission and Distribution Projects Limited)

The first interconnection between the power systems of the Central Electricity Generating Board (CEGB) in the UK and Électricité de France was completed in 1961 with the commissioning of a 160 MW, ±100 kV HVDC link between converter stations using mercury-arc valves at Lydd and Echinghen (Fig. 5.5). The cables for the link were laid directly on the sea bed and subsequently suffered damage from fishing trawls and anchors and as a result were frequently out of service. The link was finally decommissioned in 1982.

The new link is rated at 2000 MV, ±270 kV and uses air-cooled thyristor valves in its converter stations at Sellindge near Ashford in Kent and Les Mandarins in France, including a 45 km submarine crossing of the Channel (Fig. 5.5). By burying the cables in trenches on the seabed damage should be minimized, enabling the design availability of 95% to be achieved.

> Effectively two independent 1000 MW links.

The interconnection of the power systems of the UK and France has a number of features. Firstly, there is an increased diversity of availability of generating plant, with plant in one country available to support the other. The different patterns of demand can also be exploited, leading to more efficient plant operation while the country with higher marginal generating costs in any period can buy and import power from the other at lower cost.

The Scheme

The Sellindge converter station occupies a 34-acre site on the route of the Dungeness/Canterbury 400 kV transmission line. From Sellindge the cables run to Folkestone and then across the Channel to the French coast at Sangatte and on to Les Mandarins.

> Between 150 and 200 acres would have been required for an equivalent, conventional power station.

In the UK, the land cables are of the oil pressure impregnated paper type, unarmoured with a conductor cross-section of 800 mm² and an overall diameter of 80 mm. The eight cables are laid in pairs in 1.0 m deep trenches.

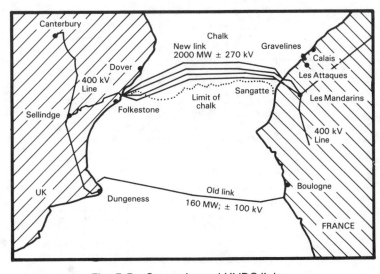

Fig. 5.5 Cross channel HVDC links.

The submarine cables are shared by the UK and France with each country providing four cables. The UK cables are of the mass impregnated solid type with a conductor cross-section of 900 mm² and an overall diameter of 105 mm. Electrical insulation is by means of 220 impregnated paper tapes wound helically over the stranded copper conductors. The cable is protected by lead and polythene sheaths and armoured with 5 mm steel wires and is manufactured in 4 × 50 km continuous lengths.

The cables are laid as four independent pairs spaced 1 km apart on the seabed. Each pair consists of a positive and a negative cable laid in a 1.5 m deep trench cut in the chalk of the seabed. The pairs are laid touching in the trench to eliminate magnetic field effects which could interfere with ships' compasses.

The UK cables are laid in a two-stage process. In the first stage an unmanned, tracked, self-propelled trenching machine is used to cut a 1.5 m deep by 0.6 m wide trench. At the same time a guide hawser is laid in the trench by the machine. Once the trench was completed the cable laying and embedding machine (CLEM) could begin installing the cables. This machine, operated from the cable laying vessel, used the previously installed guide cable to pull itself along the trench, clearing the way with high pressure water jets. The two cables are fed down to the CLEM which positions them in the trench, at the same time the guide hawser is recovered to the surface. Backfilling of the trench is then by natural movement of the bottom sediment.

The converter station

Each country assumed the responsibility for the design and construction of its own converter station, with GEC Transmission and Distribution Projects the main electrical contractor for the UK terminal at Sellindge. The general circuit for Sellindge is shown in Fig. 5.6. Because of the space restrictions on the site, metal-clad SF$_6$ switchgear is used for the 400 kV substation. Each bipole of the HVDC link is configured to be switched separately at 400 kV, as is the reactive com-

The RTM III trenching machine was developed by Land and Marine Engineering.

The CLEM was developed by Balfour Kirkpatrick.

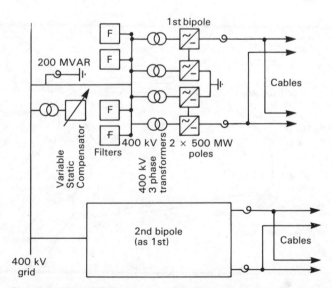

Fig. 5.6 Simplified circuit of Sellindge converter station.

pensation and auxiliary supplies. The harmonic filters are switched at the bipole 400 kV busbars.

The twelve thyristor valves that make up each 500 MW pole use air-cooled thyristors and are arranged in three, four-unit combinations referred to as quadrivalves. Each thyristor valve consists of 125 modules connected in series, a total of 6000 modules for the complete station. The modules themselves comprise a pair of parallel-connected thyristors 56 mm in diameter together with the components for the control of current and voltage stresses. The thyristors have a forward voltage capability of 3.2 kV and a reverse breakdown voltage of 4 kV. The current rating of the pair is 2000 A when operated in a full-wave bridge configuration. The nominal bridge rating is 135 kV and 1850 A using 125 series-connected modules.

See page 118 for definition of the term 'thyristor valve'. The converter station consists of a total of 48 thyristor valves arranged to form 12 quadrivalves.

The thyristors are of an established design using an inert-gas-filled, hermetically sealed capsule construction with double-sided cooling. An amplifying gate is incorporated to minimize gate power requirements. The gate signals for the valves are produced by a twelve-pulse, equidistant-firing control system and transmitted to the module using fibre optic light guides.

See Fig. 1.14(b) for details of the capsule construction of thyristors.

When operating at full rated power each thyristor valve will have a loss of less than 200 kW, giving a total loss below 4.5 MW for each bipole. Each module has its pair of thyristors mounted on copper heat sinks and these, together with the main power connections, provide the outward heat transfer. The heat output from the valves is removed by a closed-cycle, filtered air system designed to provide cooling air at an input temperature of 40°C. The heated air is cooled by an air-to-water heat exchanger with final rejection to atmosphere by spray-type cooling towers.

Instead of the conventional series-tuned filters for the control of characteristic harmonics there is a series of eight filters which will be switched in combinations determined by loading. Second-order filters will be used to control characteristic harmonics with third-order filters introduced to improve the intrinsic damping of the AC system at low frequencies and to limit non-characteristic harmonics.

See Chapter 6.

The Sellindge converter terminal will require some dynamic compensation to provide both reactive power absorbtion and generation to maintain operation at or near to unity power factor. A reactive overload absorbtion capability also is required to contain temporary overvoltages that might occur when the link is blocked, as for example following a fault, before the filters are disconnected. Two high-speed compensators are being installed at Sellindge. These are of the saturated reactor type and together with switched shunt capacitance provide ± 300 MVAR of compensation. In addition, during overloads the saturated reactors can each absorb 495 MVAR for 0.5 s. A third, identical compensator is being installed on the 400 kV system at Ninfield near Hastings to provide support to the system west of Dungeness.

Control

The link can be controlled from either of the converter stations or, more usually, the grid control centres in the UK or France. Communication between the converter stations is by power line carrier over the eight DC cables. Converter control signals are transmitted at 1200 baud and instructions and signalling at 300 baud.

(Based on: Yates, J.B. and Arnold, R. (1985). Demand patterns make submarine cross channel link economic. *Modern Power Systems*, February.)

Goddard, S.C., Yates, J.B., Urwin, R.J., le Du, A., Marechal, P. and Michel, R. (1980). The new 2000 MW interconnection between France and the United Kingdom. *International Conference on Large High Voltage Electric Systems*, CIGRE, Paper 14–09.

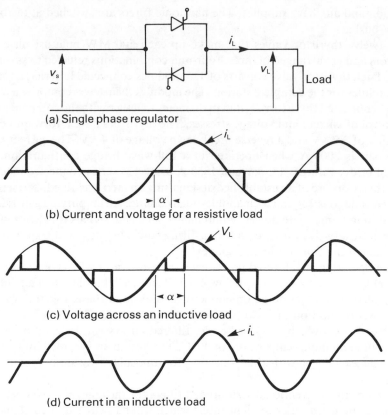

(a) Single phase regulator

(b) Current and voltage for a resistive load

(c) Voltage across an inductive load

(d) Current in an inductive load

Fig. 5.7   Single phase regulator with resistive and inductive loads.

Voltage Regulation

By connecting a reverse parallel pair of thyristors or a triac in the AC supply line the voltage supply to the load can be controlled. Figure 5.7 shows a single-phase regulator operating with both resistive and inductive loads.

With an inductive load there is a minimum firing angle determined by the phase angle of the load.

    Three-phase loads can be controlled by either of the circuits of Fig. 5.8. For the fully-controlled circuit of Fig. 5.8(a), two thyristors must always be conducting. In order to ensure that this condition exists, the thyristors must receive a second gate pulse 60° after the initial pulse, which also covers those conditions where the current is discontinuous. The actual load waveforms depend on the number of devices conducting at any instant.

    If one device in each line is conducting then operation is as for a normal three-phase system. When only two devices are conducting then the load is receiving effectively a single-phase supply and the third terminal assumes a potential which is the mean of the two conducting phase voltages. Applications of this form of control include incandescent lighting and heating.

Heating loads

A resistive load such as that used for heating can be controlled by any of the circuits of Fig. 5.7 and 5.8. The mean voltage at the load can be varied by altering the firing

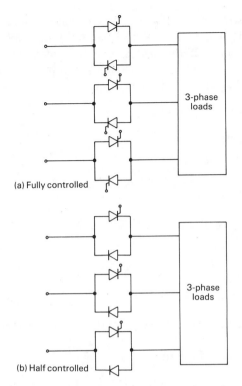

(a) Fully controlled

(b) Half controlled

Fig. 5.8   Regulators supplying three phase loads.

angle for each half cycle (*phase angle control*) as in Fig. 5.7. For a resistive load the RMS load voltage is then:

$$V_{load} = \left[\frac{1}{\pi} \int_{\alpha}^{\pi} (V_{max} \sin \theta)^2 \, d\theta \right]^{\frac{1}{2}}$$
$$= V_{max} [(\pi - \alpha + \tfrac{1}{2} \sin 2\alpha)/2\pi]^{\frac{1}{2}} \qquad (5.2)$$

This gives a load power of:

$$P_{load} = V_{max}^2 (\pi - \alpha + \tfrac{1}{2} \sin 2\alpha)/2\pi R \qquad (5.3)$$

Alternatively, where the thermal time constant is sufficiently long, the load power can be controlled by switching the supply to the load for an integral number of cycles or half cycles and then off for a further integral number of cycles or half cycles as in Fig. 5.9. The power in the load is then:

Integral cycle control or burst firing.

$$P_{load} = \frac{V_{load}^2}{R} \, \frac{N}{N + M} \qquad (5.4)$$

where N is the number of half cycles during which the supply is connected to the load and M the number of half cycles over which the supply is disconnected from the load.

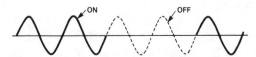

Fig. 5.9   Integral cycle control.

123

Worked Example 5.1   A single-phase resistive heating load is to be controlled from a single-phase, 50 Hz AC supply by means of an inverse parallel pair of thyristors. What will be the firing angle of the thyristors when the load is 60% of its maximum value? If this controller is replaced by a burst firing system operating with a constant repetition period of 0.24 s, what will be the range of output powers available?

From Equation 5.2

$$P_{max} = V_{max}{}^2/(2R)$$

Hence

$$\frac{P_{load}}{P_{max}} = (\pi - \alpha + \tfrac{1}{2}\sin 2\alpha)/\pi$$

When $P_{load} = 0.6P_{max}$

$$0.6 = (\pi - \alpha + \tfrac{1}{2}\sin 2\alpha)/\pi$$

Solving numerically gives

Firing angle $\alpha = 80°\ 55'$

For burst firing, the repetition frequency of 0.24 s represents 12 cycles at 50 Hz or 24 half-cycles.

Therefore, referring to Equation 5.3

$$N + M = 24$$

and

$$\frac{P_{load}}{P_{max}} = N/(N + M) = N/24$$

Available powers range from 4.17% of P_{max} ($N = 1$) to 100% of P_{max} ($N = 24$), varying in steps of 4.17% of P_{max}.

Tap-changers

Figure 5.10(a) shows a simple thyristor tap-changer providing two levels of output voltage. Provided that the firing of the thyristors is synchronized to the voltage and current this circuit will not reduce the power factor nor generate any harmonics. By varying the firing angle of the thyristors between the two pairs, additional control of the output voltage can be achieved as shown in Fig. 5.10(b). Where a greater range of variation in the output voltage is required then the arrangement of Fig. 5.10(c) could be used. By grading the secondary winding voltages and switching them in combination, a wide range of output voltages can be achieved.

Thyristor circuit Breakers

Currently, DC high-speed circuit breakers (HSCBs) are used for the protection of systems such as railway DC supplies and high-voltage DC motors. HSCBs are mechanical devices and suffer from a number of disadvantages. In particular,

Bird, B.M. and King, K.G. (1983). *An Introduction to Power Electronics*. John Wiley, U.K.

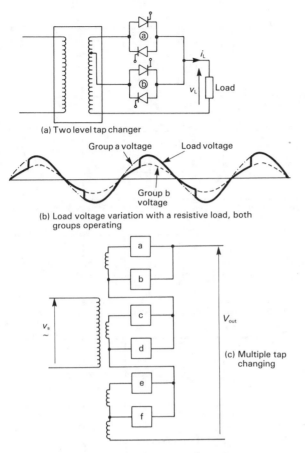

(a) Two level tap changer

(b) Load voltage variation with a resistive load, both groups operating

(c) Multiple tap changing

Fig. 5.10   Thyristor tap changers.

contacts are eroded by the switching of load currents and operation against faults, creating maintainance problems, operating speed may be inadequate to provide proper protection to semiconductor devices and the high temperature of the arcs on fault interruption creates problems of heat removal. The thyristor DC circuit breaker is a method of providing a fast, static means of interrupting DC current which is capable of repeated operation with low maintainance.

The principle of operation of the thyristor DC circuit breaker is shown by Fig. 5.11. In normal operation the current path is as in Fig. 5.11(a). When the fault occurs the rise in the current through the main thyristor is detected and the auxiliary thyristor turned on, discharging the capacitor through the main thyristor to commutate it off. This condition is shown in Fig. 5.11(b). The current path is now via the auxiliary thyristor as in Fig. 5.11(c) and the capacitor charges in the reverse direction causing the auxiliary thyristor to turn-off when the current through it falls below its holding level. Energy in the load inductance is then dissipated by the circulating current in the freewheeling diode as in Fig. 5.11(d).

See Chapter 3 for forced commutation circuits.

Table 5.1 sets out some of the stages in the development of thyristor circuit breakers. The majority of thyristor circuit breaker applications to date have been on railway traction systems where their capacity for repeated operation, low main-

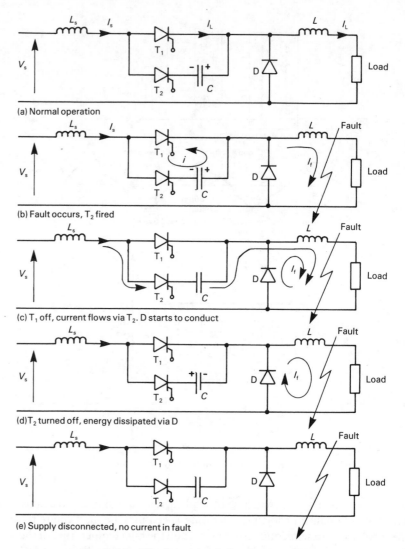

(a) Normal operation

(b) Fault occurs, T_2 fired

(c) T_1 off, current flows via T_2. D starts to conduct

(d) T_2 turned off, energy dissipated via D

(e) Supply disconnected, no current in fault

Fig. 5.11   Thyristor circuit breaker operation.

tainance costs and the ability to dissipate the energy in the catenary system offset the increase in cost relative to mechanical HSCBs.

Power supplies

Switched-mode Power Supplies

Though the switched-mode power supply (SMPS) was developed originally by NASA in the 1960s to provide a compact power-supply system for space vehicles it did not have a significant impact on the general power supply market until the 1970s. From that point development was rapid and the SMPS now accounts for some 70% of the power supplies being produced.

A SMPS is based on a DC chopper with a rectified and possibly transformed

Cuk, S. (May, 1984). Survey of switched mode power supplies. IEE Conference Publication 234, *Power Electronics and Variable Speed Drives*, pp. 83–94.

Table 5.1 Development of Thyristor Circuit-breakers
(Dr P. McEwan, personal communication)

Thyristor circuit-breaker	Rated voltage (V)	Rated current (A)	Trip setting (A)	Peak let-through current (A)	Operating time (ms)	Application
Goldberg (1963)	120	5	12	25	0.04	Inverse time overload and short-circuit protection.
Zyborski (1976)	600	800	500 to 1500	1850	1.02	Overcurrent protection. Gdansk trolley-bus system.
Zyborski (1980)	1000		2700	3400	4	Experimental switch for overcurrent protection.
Modified Mazda (1982)	110		80	100	1.4	Experimental switch for low voltage DC with auto reclose.
Mitsubishi (1982)	1500	1300	4500	9700	< 10	Kotoni traction system, Sapporo.
Meidenisha (1982)	1500		3000	4200		Tozai subway line, Sapporo
Toshiba (1982)	1500	3000	6000	7500	2.9	Teito Rapid Transit Authority.

output. The output voltage amplitude is controlled by varying the mark–space ratio of the chopper. This may be achieved by means of pulse-width control or frequency variation with constant pulse width, the former being the more common. The circuit techniques used for SMPS can be separated into four broad categories — flyback, feed-forward, push-pull and bridge.

See Chapter 3 for chopper operation.

Figure 5.12(a) shows a simplified circuit for a single transistor flyback SMPS. During the conduction period of the transistor the current in the inductance varies such that

$$L\Delta i_1 = V_s\Delta t = V_s\delta T \qquad (5.5)$$

where T is $1/f$ and f is the switching frequency
and $\quad \Delta t = \delta T$ is the period for which the transistor is conducting.
$\quad\quad\quad \delta$ therefore has a value between 0 and 1.

When the transistor stops conducting, energy is transferred from the magnetic field

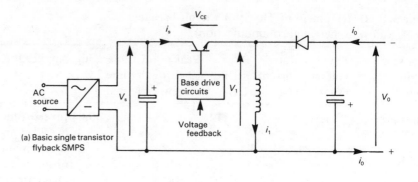

(a) Basic single transistor flyback SMPS

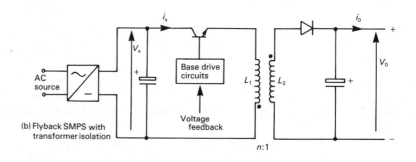

(b) Flyback SMPS with transformer isolation

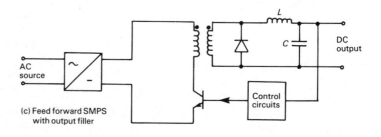

(c) Feed forward SMPS with output filler

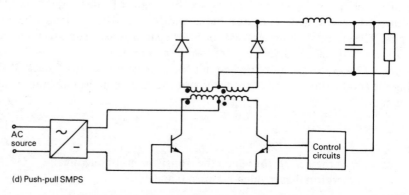

(d) Push-pull SMPS

Fig. 5.12: Types of switched mode power supply.

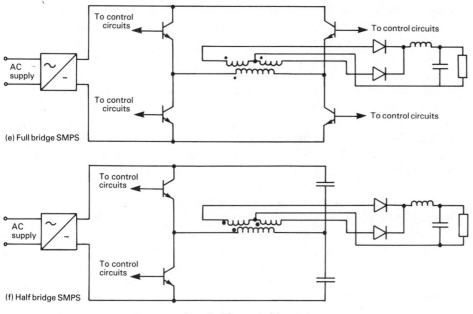

(e) Full bridge SMPS

(f) Half bridge SMPS

Fig. 5.12   cont'd

of the inductive choke to the load via the diode. The change in the current during this period is

$$L\Delta i_1 = V_0(1 - \delta)T \qquad (5.6)$$

At equilibrium, the change in current magnitude is the same during both the conducting and non-conducting periods. Equations 5.5 and 5.6 can therefore be combined to give

$$V_0 = \frac{V_s\delta}{(1 - \delta)} \qquad (5.7)$$

For this relationship to be valid the magnitude of the ripple current must not affect the conduction period of the thyristor. The inductance L is therefore chosen to limit the maximum value of the ripple current to twice the average value of the minimum choke current. Now

$$I_{1,\text{mean}} = \frac{I_{0,\text{mean}}}{(1 - \delta)} \qquad (5.8)$$

Hence, referring to Equation 5.6, the minimum value for L can be obtained:

$$L_{\min} = \left(\frac{V_s V_0}{V_3 + V_0}\right)^2 \frac{T}{2P_0}$$

where $P_0 = V_0 I_{0,\text{mean}}$; the output power.

The magnitude of the output voltage can be controlled and isolation provided for the output by adding a second winding to the choke to form a transformer as in Fig. 5.12(b). In this case the value V_0 in Equations 5.5 to 5.9 is replaced by nV_0, where n is the transformer turns ratio, and L by L_1.

Though using a minimal number of components the simple flyback SMPS makes inefficient use of the transistor and generates relatively high levels of noise in its output. Therefore applications tend to be limited to power levels of the order of a few hundred watts.

The feed-forward arrangement of Fig. 5.12(c) uses an output filter to store energy during the off period and this energy is fed to the load via the commutating diode. This results in a reduction in the ripple in the final output voltage.

The push-pull configuration of Fig. 5.12(d) offers higher efficiency but suffers from the fact that the transistors can experience voltages up to twice the DC input voltage as a result of transformer action. Bridges can be either full (Fig. 5.12(e)) or half (Fig. 5.12(f)) with the highest efficiency and best output performance achieved by the full-bridge.

The overall size of a SMPS is a function of frequency with operation commonly in the range 20 to 50 kHz. For operation at frequencies of 100 kHz and higher use is being made of power MOS devices to handle the high switching rates.

A comparison between a conventional, linear power supply and a SMPS shows that for the same output rating a SMPS will be of smaller size, lighter weight and higher efficiency. It will also be less sensitive to variations in its input voltage. On the debit side, the SMPS has a higher output ripple and its regulation is likely to be worse, as is its dynamic response. The SMPS is also a source of both electromagnetic and radio frequency interference which may appear in the AC supply, as radiated noise or in the output. Control of these various forms of noise is achieved by filtering on both the input and output of the SMPS and by careful screening and attention to the layout of the circuit board.

Case Study — Television Receiver Power Supply
(Mullard Ltd)

A television receiver is very sensitive to variations in the voltage supply to its deflection circuits, relatively small changes in these voltages being reflected in visible changes in picture size. For this reason the SMPS with its ability to provide a stable output voltage over a wide range of loads and input voltage conditions has been adopted for use in television receiver horizontal deflection circuits.

The variation of picture size due to variations in voltage amplitude is referred to as 'picture breathing'.

Figure 5.13 shows the block diagram of a SMPS supplying the horizontal deflection circuit, east-west raster correction circuit, line deflection coil, sound output stage and some auxiliary circuits. The SMPS is of the single transistor flyback type and has the performance requirements set out in Table 5.2.

The design of the SMPS must be such as to ensure that the operating load line of the output switching transistor is maintained within its SOAR under all operating conditions. Additionally, action must be taken to prevent any radio frequency interference (RFI) generated by the SMPS causing visible interference on the screen. Referring to the SMPS output circuit of Fig. 5.14 the RFI can be controlled by the connection of the output switching transistor to the upper end of the transformer primary and by the inclusion of capacitor C_1. The first of these measures maintains the stray capacitance at the collector of the output switching transistor at a constant potential, reducing switching spikes, while the inclusion of C_1 reduces the dV/dt values and minimizes the length of the radiation loop.

Further measures required to maintain the output switching transistor within its

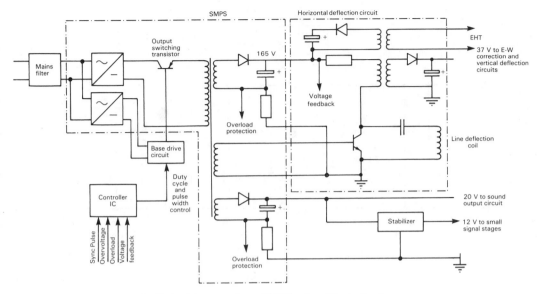

Fig. 5.13   Television receiver SMPS, simplified circuit.

Table 5.2   Requirements of Switched-mode Power Supply for Television Receiver

Mains voltage range	V_{mains}	187–265 V AC (220 V, $+20\%$, -15%)
Main output voltage	V_0	165 V DC
Minimum load on main output	$P_{0,min}$	60 W
Maximum load on main output	$P_{0,max}$	120 W
Losses in SMPS output circuit	P_{loss}	10 W
Minimum auxiliary load	$P_{a,min}$	10 W
Maximum auxiliary load	$P_{a,max}$	20 W
Base drive auxiliary load	P_{drive}	4 W
Stabilization of main output		Better than 3%
Ripple level 50/100 Hz hum		Less than 0.2%
Switching frequency		15 625 Hz ($T = 64$ μs)

SOAR are the inclusion of the inductance L to limit the peak current in C_1 on turn-on, the addition of the D_1–R_1 combination to damp out the LC_1 oscillations and the inclusion of capacitor C_2 to minimize the peak voltage across the transistor by passing the peak current. Finally, the D_2–R_2–C_3 network is incorporated to limit overshoot due to the transformer leakage inductance on turn-off.

The base drive to the output switching transistor provides a fast rising base current for rapid turn-on to minimize switching losses. Following turn-on the transistor is maintained in saturation for the duration of its conduction period. Losses on turn-off are minimized by ensuring that a reverse base current is maintained once the collector current starts to decrease. The base drive circuit must also be able to hold the output switching transistor off following remote turn-off or operation of protection systems. It also provides the interface between the control circuits and the output switching transistor.

Overload protection is provide in each of the output transformer secondaries by

See Chapter 1 for discussion of transistor turn-on and turn-off.

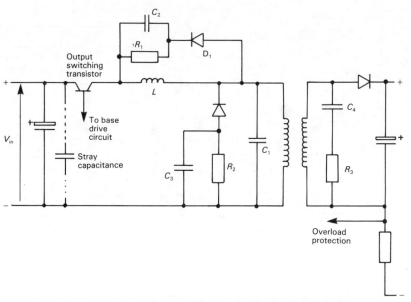

Fig. 5.14 Television receiver SMPS, control circuits to maintain output transistor within its SOAR.

sensing the voltage across a reference resistor connected to earth. This voltage is taken to the controller integrated circuit which will then shut down the SMPS on detecting an overload condition. The collector current of the output switching transistor can be measured directly by including a current-sensing transformer in series with the transistor. The output from this transformer is converter to a voltage signal and taken to the overvoltage detection circuit of the controller integrated circuit.

The operation of the SMPS can result in the following types of interference:

(a) *Visible interference* — the result of spurious radiated signals into the tuner and/or i.f. amplifiers of the receiver. The principal source of this interference is the high di/dt of the current pulse produced by the output switching transistor.
(b) *Symmetrical mains pollution* — caused by the SMPS switching the current drawn through the main input rectifier.
(c) *Asymmetrical mains pollution* — appears between the earth and the supply line and neutral conductors. Its source is the capacitive currents flowing between the high level AC voltages and earth.

In addition to the measures already described for the limitation of visible interference caused by RFI, further control can be achieved by:

(a) Limiting the dV/dt in the rectifiers in the output transformer secondaries by the connection of a capacitor in parallel with the rectifier diode.
(b) Decreasing the dV/dt in the base drive transistor by means of an RC network in the collector of the output switching transistor.
(c) Providing a low-inductance path from the common line on the mains isolated side of the supply to the receiver chassis.

The mains interference can be controlled by:

(a) The inclusion of filtering in the mains input lines.
(b) Shielding the transformer to prevent stray voltages.
(c) Connection of a small capacitor (<4.7 nF) between the mains isolated and non-isolated common rails.

The controller integrated circuit is a single-chip system which provides all the control functions for the SMPS. These include:

(a) Control of the duty cycle of the output switching transistor to compensate for variations in the load and supply voltage.
(b) Overcurrent protection incorporating automatic restart after a transient fault.
(c) Overvoltage protection.
(d) Slow-start to limit the inrush currents on turn-on and including protection against a fault in the feedback loop during the start-up sequence.
(e) Protection against low supply voltage and against a disconnected or open circuit voltage reference diode.
(f) A rapid response control loop to compensate for delays in the horizontal deflection circuit. This enables the horizontal deflection drive to be obtained from the SMPS.

(Based on: SMPS in tv receivers — Circuits with mains isolation. *Mullard Technical Information No 49*. Reproduced by permission of Mullard Ltd.)

Series-resonant power supply

The basic series-resonant power supply (SRPS) is shown in Fig. 5.15. By switching the GTO thyristor the series-resonant LC circuit is maintained in oscillation producing a sinusoidal output voltage V_0.

Consider the unloaded circuit of Fig. 5.15, as $L_2 \gg L_1$ its influence on operation can be ignored. Initially with the GTO off, C_1 is charged to the supply voltage. If the GTO is now turned on just long enough to discharge C_1, then, when the GTO is turned off, the current i_1 oscillates relative to zero at a frequency set by L_1 together with C_1 and C_0 in series.

Nijhof E.B.G. and Evers, H.W. (November 1981). Introduction to the series-resonant power supply. *Electronic Components and Applications* **4** (1).

L_2 should be a minimum of 10 L_1 and C_0 should be at least twice C_1.

$$\omega = 1/\sqrt{(L_1 C_x)} \qquad (5.10)$$

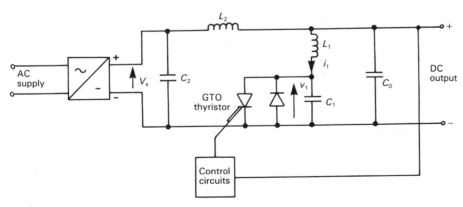

Fig. 5.15 Basic circuit of a SRPS.

where

$$C_x = C_1 C_0 / (C_1 + C_0) \tag{5.11}$$

For stable self-oscillation V_1 must reach zero during each cycle. V_1 is given by:

$$V_1 = V_s(1 - \cos \omega t) \tag{5.12}$$

and varies between 0 and $2V_s$. The output voltage is determined by the values of C_1 and C_0. The peak value of V_0 is:

$$V_{0,max} = V_s(C_1 + C_0) / C_0 \tag{5.13}$$

and has an AC component of amplitude

$$V_{0,AC} = V_s C_1 / C_0 \tag{5.14}$$

If the conduction period of the GTO is increased, current will be flowing in L_1 on turn-off resulting in an increase in the peak oscillatory current by an amount

$$N = (I_x Z_1 / V_s)^2 + 1 \tag{5.15}$$

This results in an AC output voltage amplitude of

$$V_{0,AC} = NV_s C_1 / C_0 \tag{5.16}$$

This means that control of the output voltage can be achieved by varying the conduction period of the GTO. Depending on the circuit conditions multiplying factors (N) of 11 can be achieved and the output stabilized against input voltage variations of 6 to 1.

Power can be taken from the SRPS in a number of ways, some of which are shown in Fig. 5.16. In Fig. 5.16(a) the connection is via a diode to a smoothing

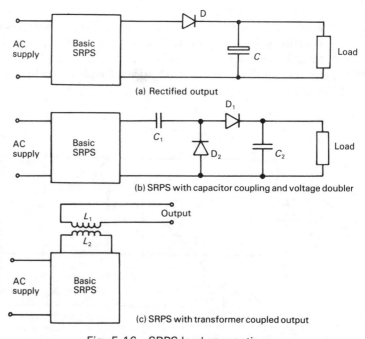

(a) Rectified output

(b) SRPS with capacitor coupling and voltage doubler

(c) SRPS with transformer coupled output

Fig. 5.16   SRPS load connections.

capacitor and the load. Used in this way the SRPS can be arranged to supply a stabilized output voltage with a small ripple at twice the supply frequency. No smoothing is required on the input rectifier, reducing the harmonic currents fed back into the supply.

If instead a capacitor-coupled output is used, an AC signal at the oscillatory frequency is available at the output. This signal could be used either directly or via circuits such as the voltage doubler of Fig. 5.16(b).

In Fig. 5.16(c) the output is transformer coupled with inductance L_2 incorporated into the transformer inductance. This enables the load to be matched to the SRPS by varying the turns ratio. This gives good mains isolation and can be used to supply resistive or rectifier loads. A further modification incorporates inductance L_1 within the transformer. In this form the SRPS is inherently immune to a short-circuited output and is self-starting under all conditions.

Uninterruptable power supplies

In applications such as hospital intensive care systems, chemical plant process control, safety monitors or a major computer installation, where even a temporary loss of supply could have severe consequences, there is a need to provide an uninterruptable power supply (UPS) system which can maintain the supply under all conditions.

Initially, UPS systems were based on arrangements of the type shown in Fig. 5.17 where a DC motor is used to drive an AC generator, the shaft of which is also coupled to a diesel engine. On failure of the mains supply the diesel engine was started and took over the load after a delay of 10 to 15 seconds. By incorporating into the system a flywheel together with a battery supply to the DC motor, the generator speed can largely be maintained during the start-up of the diesel engine, to give a no-break supply.

Static UPS systems operate by rectifying the incoming AC supply and using this voltage to feed an inverter which then supplies the load. In the case of a failure of the AC supply, the supply to the inverter is taken over by a battery bank, supplemented in some cases by a standby DC generator driven by a diesel engine to cover a long-duration failure of the main AC supply.

Figure 5.18 shows two forms of static UPS system. In the configuration of

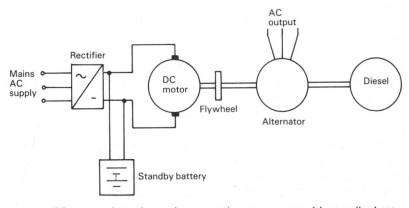

Fig. 5.17 UPS system based on a d.c. motor/generator set with standby battery and diesel prime mover.

The battery-charging circuit would normally be arranged to provide a continuous trickle charging current to the batteries.

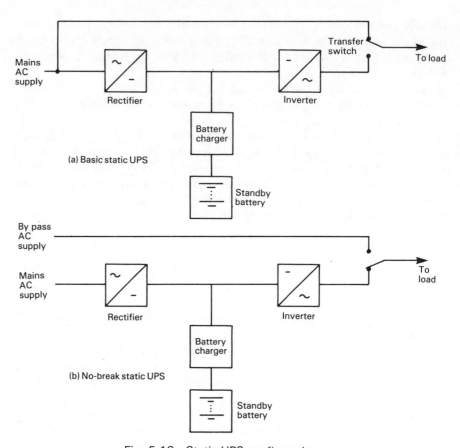

(a) Basic static UPS

(b) No-break static UPS

Fig. 5.18   Static UPS configurations.

Fig. 5.18(a) the load is normally supplied from the main AC supply with the rectifier maintaining the batteries on full charge. In the event of supply failure the load is switched on to the output of the inverter which then takes over supply. Where a no-break supply is required the arrangement of Fig. 5.18(b) is used in which normally the load is connected to the output of the inverter and the rectifier both supplies the inverter and maintains the charge on the standby batteries. This configuration has the added advantage that the inverter can be used to condition the supply to the load, to protect the load from transients in the main AC supply and to maintain the load frequency within preset limits. As in this mode the inverter is in continuous operation, provision must be made in case of its failure. This is done by switching the load to the main AC supply should inverter failure be detected. By using a solid-state switch this transfer can be achieved in 4 to 5 ms as opposed to some 40 or 50 ms for a mechanical contactor.

Typical installations would use either nickel–cadmium or lead–acid batteries to provide the back-up. Nickel–cadmium batteries have the advantages that their electrolyte is non-corrosive, do not emit an explosive gas when charging and they cannot be damaged by overcharging or discharging. Their cost, however, is two to three times that of lead–acid batteries. The length of time the inverter can be supported by the batteries depends on the size of the batteries and the nature of the load.

A solid-state switch is made up of a pair of thyristors in reverse parallel. When the switch is ON these are fired at zero delay.

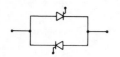

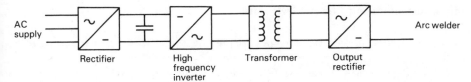

Fig. 5.19 Arc welder using an inverter power supply.

Once the main supply has been restored the batteries are recharged from the main supply. This is normally done by operating the charger at maximum charge rate to ensure that fully battery capacity is restored as quickly as possible.

Welding

A conventional DC arc welding system requires a high current at a voltage in the range 50–100 V. This step-down is provided by the large, heavy and expensive mains transformer which also provides the necessary isolation between the incoming supply and the welding arc. By increasing the transformer operating frequency a smaller transformer can be used since for the same working flux density and output voltage a smaller cross-sectional area of core is required at the higher frequency.

A welding supply operating on this principle is shown in Fig. 5.19. The incoming AC supply is first rectified and used as the supply to a high-frequency inverter, the output of which is connected via a transformer and rectifier to supply the arc. By using asymmetric and GTO thyristors, supplies with ratings of 15 kVA at frequencies of 30 kHz are achievable at efficiencies of the order of 80 to 85%.

Compared with 50% or less for a conventional welding supply.

Estimate the change in core cross-section required between ideal transformers of the same ratio and with the same maximum core flux density operating at frequencies of 50 Hz and 20 kHz.

Worked Example 5.2

Let $\phi = \phi_{max} \sin \omega t$
and $e_a = N d\phi/dt = \omega N \phi_{max} \cos \omega t$
Hence $E_{a,RMS} = \omega N \phi_{max}/\sqrt{2}$
For constant $E_{a,RMS}$

$$\phi_{max} \propto 1/\omega$$

Now

$$\phi_{max} = B_{max} \times \text{(core cross-sectional area)}$$

Therefore, for constant B_{max}

Core cross-sectional area $\propto 1/\omega$
$$\frac{\text{Core cross-section at 50 Hz}}{\text{Core cross-section at 20000 Hz}} = 400{:}1$$

Microelectronics and Power Electronics

Microprocessors and microelectronics are playing a significant and expanding role in the real-time control of power electronic systems ranging from variable-speed drives to power transmission, resulting in increased performance and efficiency by optimization of system operation. Where a single processor is used for this purpose, then its interrupt structure becomes important along with the assignment of priorities within the system. However, with the reduction in the cost of microprocessors there is an increasing tendency towards the distribution of intelligence throughout a system with individual microprocessors allocated to the control of specific functions within the overall system. These developments, together with the ability of the microprocessor to handle complex algorithms, have increased operational flexibility and enabled system characteristics to be more closely matched to load requirements. These conditions are of particular importance where a number of functions such as the individual joint movements of a robot or the drive rollers of a paper mill need to be co-ordinated.

In applications where speed of operation is a significant factor the programs for the microprocessor would be written in the assembly language of the particular processor. Such an approach, while providing programs which are fast and of minimum size, is expensive in development time. By writing in a high-level language, software costs are reduced at the expense of a less efficient program. As a compromise, the bulk of the program may be written in the high-level language, using the assembly language only for the time-critical areas.

Since the introduction of the first microprocessors the developments in manufacturing technology have resulted in devices with architectures ranging from 4 to 32 bits. These are supported by an increasing range of single-chip microprocessors and microcontrollers. For applications involving high production volumes these single-chip devices provide a cost-effective approach to hardware.

Single-chip microcontrollers have been developed specifically for control applications and incorporate timers, counters, analogue-to-digital converters, input/output structures and RAM and ROM memory on the same chip. Future developments are likely to involve the incorporation of some of the following features on to the single-chip device:

Improved processor architecture
Increased on-board RAM and ROM
Enhanced input/output (I/O) facilities
Memory Management Units
Hardware multiply/divide
Enhanced timers
Watchdog timers
Phase-locked loops
Improved analogue-to-digital and digital-to-analogue converters
Multiplexers and comparators
Signal generators
Communications controllers

This list is by no means comprehensive but serves to illustrate the directions taken by the single-chip microprocessors and microcontrollers.

A natural development is the use of custom-designed and manufactured integrated circuits taking account of the improvements in device technologies and manufacturing techniques. When used in combination with power semiconductors such circuits form the basis of 'smart power' devices. These will carry on board the necessary I/O for both control and status information, isolation, required intelligence and logic, protection, packaged power supplies and device drive circuits. Manufacture could either be as a monolithic integration with all functions incorporated on a single chip or in a hybrid form with separate logic and power chips.

Applications for custom integrated circuits include the production of the switching sequence for stepper motors or the generation of inverter PWM waveforms for AC motor control. Smart power devices would include intelligent switches capable of monitoring and reporting their own status, incorporation within the housing of a stepper motor to control operation or, with appropriate communications included, a part of a network structure integrating a number of systems.

Case Study — Microeletronic Motor Speed Controller
(Polkinghorne Industries)

Series universal motors up to 750 W (1HP) rating and running at speeds up to 12 000 r/min are used in a wide range of domestic appliances such as automatic washing machines, duplicators, food mixers, portable drilling machines and saw benches. The requirements for the associated motor controller are low cost, high reliability and ease of application. By designing and developing their own integrated circuits, Polkinghornes have developed a controller module for motors of this type with around 40 components, significantly less than the discrete component equivalent. This reduced number of components not only produces a significant price reduction but also means fewer connections on the printed circuit board, leading to a more reliable unit.

The basic speed-control module can have many derivatives as the basic circuit design can be modified readily to suit individual needs such as the provision of current limit control and additional speed settings. For example, the module can be configured to provide a wide range of speed settings over a range of system voltages.

Various forms of protection are incorporated within the module. In the case of a tachogenerator failure, either open or short circuit, the signal from the tachogenerator is lost and the module brings the motor to zero speed rather than allowing any acceleration to a possibly hazardous condition. Should the motor become stalled for any reason the module will again shut down the power supply to prevent burn-out. Reaction in either of the above two conditions is within one second.

The module is protected against the failure of the motor triac by the use of a discrete, low-cost, sacrificial transistor which is used to drive the triac and protect the more expensive integrated circuit. Following a failure of this type the module can easily and cheaply be repaired for subsequent re-use. The drive triac is rated at 12 A at 500 V, will take an inrush current of 85 A and can withstand a stalled rotor current of 30 A for four seconds.

A necessary feature for the intended applications in domestic appliances is

The series universal or series commutator motor is a DC series motor operating from an AC supply. The action of the commutator means that the field and armature currents reverse direction together, maintaining a constant direction for torque. Motors of this type are capable of operating at high speeds.

protection against the voltage spikes associated with series commutator motors. Immunity is therefore provided against mains spikes up to 2000 V.

Features of particular interest are the provision of a soft-start facility, of particularly importance with belt drives to ensure that there is no belt slippage while accelerating in order to maximize belt life, and a programmed restart facility following power failure.

Frequency sensing is by means of a tachogenerator on the motor shaft. This enables factory presetting for multiple speed ranges such as might be used by a washing machine wash-and-spin cycle.

Problems

5.1 A bipolar HVDC transmission system is rated at 2000 MW, ± 320 kV and uses the converter arrangement of Fig. 5.3. Find the RMS current and peak reverse voltage for each of the thyristor valves.

5.2 A three-phase resistive heating load is controlled by triacs from a 415 V (line), 50 Hz supply. If the maximum load is 24 kW, determine the rating of the triacs and their firing angles for loads of 16 kW and 8 kW. If the triacs are replaced by thyristors, how would the current ratings change?

5.3 A single-phase load of resistance 12 Ω in series with an inductance of 24 mH is fed from a 240 V (RMS), 50 Hz supply by a pair of inverse parallel thyristors. Find the mean power in the load at firing angles of (a) 0°, (b) 90° and (c) 120°. Ignore source inductance and device voltage drops.

5.4 A tap changer such as that shown in Fig. 5.10 is used to supply a resistive load. If the lower taping is at 67% of full voltage, plot a curve showing the variation of the RMS voltage of the load against the firing angle of the 100% tapping thyristors.

5.5 A single transistor, flyback switched-mode power supply operating at 16 kHz is supplying a mean load power of 120 W at a mean voltage of 80 V from a DC source of 110 V. Estimate the mark/space ratio of the output voltage and the value of inductance required in the circuit.

Harmonics and Interference 6

Objectives

- ☐ To consider the representation of harmonic sources.
- ☐ To consider briefly the effect of harmonics on system components.
- ☐ To examine AC and DC system harmonics.
- ☐ To consider the harmonics produced by inverters and integral cycle controllers.
- ☐ To examine the basic techniques of harmonic filtering and to introduce filter types.
- ☐ To introduce harmonic standards.
- ☐ To consider briefly the production of radio-frequency interference

Rectifiers and converters operate by switching an AC supply to produce a DC voltage. In doing so they introduce harmonics into both the AC and DC systems. Inverters similarly switch a DC source of either current or voltage to produce an alternating, but non-sinusoidal, output which again contains harmonics.

Arrilaga, J., Bradley, D.A. and Bodger, P.S. (1985). *Power System Harmonics*. John Wiley, U.K.

Supply System Harmonics

For self-commutated converters operating from a sinusoidal voltage source the effect on the supply system can be considered as that of connecting a number of harmonic current generators feeding back into the AC system. These harmonic currents then combine with the system impedances at the harmonic frequencies to produce the harmonic voltages.

The presence of these harmonic currents and voltages can influence system behaviour in a number of ways. Among these are:

(a) Amplification of system current and voltage levels as a result of series or parallel resonances.
(b) Increased losses in system components such as generating plant, power-factor correction capacitors and motors.
(c) Ageing of insulation leading to a reduction in operational lifetimes.
(d) Plant maloperation.
(e) Interference with communications systems.

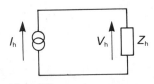

$V_h = I_h Z_h$

I_h = Harmonic current

V_h = Harmonic voltage

Z_h = Impedance at harmonic frequency

Harmonic equivalent circuit.

Figure 6.1 shows a general, ideal p-pulse converter together with a quasi square-wave representing the current waveform for one phase of the supply. The Fourier series ($F(t)$) for this waveform is:

$$F(t) = \frac{4}{\pi}\left[\sin\frac{\psi}{2}\cos(\omega t) + \frac{1}{3}\sin\frac{3\psi}{2}\cos(3\omega t)\right.$$
$$\left. + \frac{1}{5}\sin\frac{5\psi}{2}\cos(5\omega t) + \ldots\ldots\ldots\ldots \right] \tag{6.1}$$

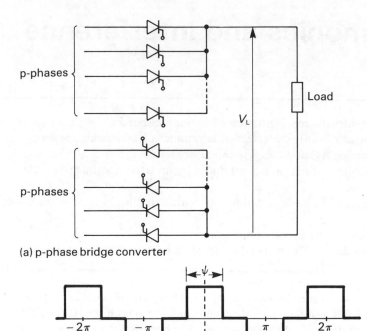

(a) p-phase bridge converter

(b) Quasi-square wave

Fig. 6.1   Operation of a general p-pulse bridge.

For an ideal six-pulse converter $\psi = 2\pi/3$ when, for a DC current amplitude of I_{DC}, the current in phase 'a' is:

$$i_a = \frac{2\sqrt{3}}{\pi} I_{DC} \left[\cos \omega t - \frac{1}{5} \cos (5\omega t) + \frac{1}{7} \cos (7\omega t) \right.$$
$$- \frac{1}{11} \cos (11\omega t) + \frac{1}{13} \cos (13\omega t) - \frac{1}{17} \cos (17\omega t)$$
$$\left. + \frac{1}{19} \cos (19\omega t) - \ldots\ldots + \ldots\ldots - \ldots\ldots \right] \tag{6.2}$$

This contains harmonics of the order $n = 6k \pm 1$, where $k = 1, 2, 3$, etc., decreasing in magnitude with respect to the fundamental by:

$$I_n = I_1/n \tag{6.3}$$

where n is the harmonic number.

Similarly, the phase current for a twelve-pulse converter can be obtained as:

$$i_a = \frac{4\sqrt{3}}{\pi} I_{DC} \left[\cos \omega t - \frac{1}{11} \cos (11\omega t) + \frac{1}{13} \cos (13\omega t) \right.$$
$$\left. - \frac{1}{23} \cos (2\omega t) + \frac{1}{25} \cos (25\omega t) - \ldots\ldots + \ldots\ldots \right] \tag{6.4}$$

This contains harmonics of the order $n = 12k \pm 1$, decreasing in magnitude according to Equation 6.3. From Equations 6.2 and 6.4 the supply system harmonic components of an ideal p-pulse converter are seen to be at orders of:

$pk \pm 1$, where p is the pulse number and $k = 1, 2, 3$, etc.

However, a real converter operates with overlap and this will cause the actual harmonic content to vary from these ideal values. Figure 6.2 shows the effect of varying both the overlap and firing angle on the system harmonic currents for various harmonics.

The curves of Fig. 6.2 are sometimes referred to as Read's curves.

For a six-pulse fully-controlled converter, estimate the total harmonic distortion of current at firing angles of 0°, 10° and 30°. How would these results be affected if the converter was operating with 15° overlap?

Worked Example 6.1

Total harmonic distortion is defined as

$$\frac{\left[\sum_{n=2}^{\infty} U_n^2\right]^{\frac{1}{2}}}{U_1}$$

(1) *Zero overlap*

$\alpha = 0°$; amplitude of fundamental current = 100%

From the curves of Fig. 6.2:

Amplitude of 5th harmonic $= I_5 = 20\%$

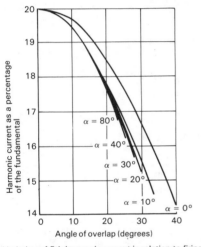

(a) Variation of 5th harmonic current in relation to firing angle and overlap angle

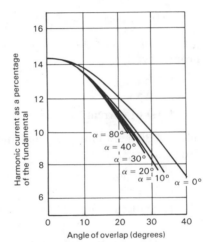

(b) Variation of 7th harmonic current in relation to firing angle and overlap angle

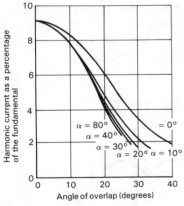

(c) Variation of 11th harmonic current in relation to firing angle and overlap angle

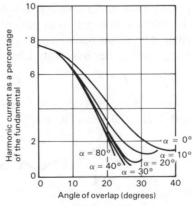

(d) Variation of 13th harmonic current in relation to firing angle and overlap angle

Fig. 6.2   Effect of firing angle and overlap on harmonic content.

Amplitude of 7th harmonic $= I_7 = 14.3\%$
Amplitude of 11th harmonic $= I_{11} = 9.1\%$
Amplitude of 13th harmonic $= I_{13} = 7.7\%$

Total harmonic distortion (THD) of current $= \dfrac{\left(\displaystyle\sum_{n=2}^{\infty} I_n^2 \right)^{1/2}}{I_1}$

$= (20^2 + 14.3^2 + 9.1^2 + 7.7^2)^{1/2} = 27.3\%$

(30% if all harmonics to 50th are included)
This result is the same for all firing angles.

(2) *15° overlap*
(i) $\alpha = 0°$; amplitude of fundamental current = 100%
From curves:

$I_5 = 19.4\%$	$I_{11} = 7.5\%$
$I_7 = 13.3\%$	$I_{13} = 5.6\%$
THD of current = 25.3%	

(ii) $\alpha = 10°$; amplitude of fundamental current = 100%
From curves:

$I_5 = 18.8\%$	$I_{11} = 6.5\%$
$I_7 = 12.8\%$	$I_{13} = 5\%$
THD of current = 24.2%	

(iii) $\alpha = 30°$; amplitude of fundamental current = 100%
From curves:

$I_5 = 18.8\%$	$I_{11} = 6.5\%$
$I_7 = 12.7\%$	$I_{13} = 4.8\%$
THD of current = 24.1%	

Dobinson, L.G. (May 1975).
Closer accord on harmonics.
Electronics and Power, 567–72.

Where there is insufficient load inductance the AC system currents may contain a significant ripple as in Fig. 6.3, or even become discontinuous. By assuming that the ripple is formed from part of a sinewave displaced relative to the zero DC current level, expressions can be obtained for the fundamental component and the characteristic harmonics in terms of the ripple factor r, where:

$$r = I_r/I_d \qquad (6.5)$$

where I_r is the peak-to-peak amplitude of the ripple current
and I_d is the mean DC current

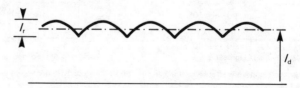

Fig. 6.3 Converter load current including ripple.

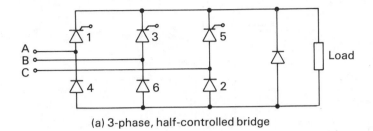

(a) 3-phase, half-controlled bridge

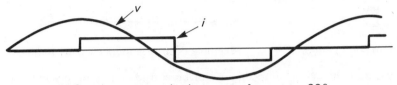

(b) Supply current and voltage waveforms, $\alpha = 60°$

Fig. 6.4   Operation of a three phase, half controlled bridge.

The fundamental component of current is given by:

$$I_1 = I_d(1.102 + 0.014r) \tag{6.6}$$

The harmonic currents, expressed as a percentage of the fundamental are then:

$$I_n = 100 \left(\frac{1}{n} + \frac{6.46r}{n-1} - \frac{7.13r}{n} \right)(-1)^k \tag{6.7}$$

for $n = kp - 1$

and

$$I_n = 100 \left(\frac{1}{n} + \frac{6.46r}{n+1} - \frac{7.13r}{n} \right)(-1)^k \tag{6.8}$$

for $n = kp + 1$

Where regeneration is not a requirement, half-controlled bridges provide a cheaper solution then the fully-controlled bridge. When operated at full voltage ($\alpha = 0°$), the harmonic currents produced by a half-controlled bridge correspond to those of the fully-controlled bridge at full voltage. However, as firing angle is increased the current waveform loses its half-wave symmetry, as is shown by Fig. 6.4. Under these conditions the half-controlled bridge can generate high levels of harmonic current and under very light load conditions a second harmonic component can result whose amplitude approaches that of the fundamental.

Full output voltage is obtained for a firing angle of 0° ($\alpha = 0°$).

Worked Example 6.2

In the system shown, consumer A has a connected load of 380 kVA at a power factor of 0.95 lagging and wishes to connect a variable-speed AC drive using an uncontrolled six-pulse converter at the 11 kV busbar. The full-load fundamental current of the converter is measured at 4.2 A/phase and it operates with a 10° overlap angle. Consumer B has a normal connected load of 485.3 kVA at a power factor of 0.75 lagging and has installed 247.1 kVA of power factor correction capacitors at the busbar.

The system fault level at the 11 kV busbar, including the transformer, is

145

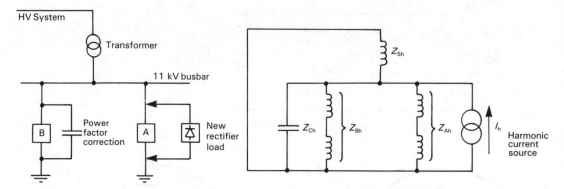

Example 6.2a   System configuration.   Example 6.2b   Harmonic system model.

30 MVA and the system impedance can be considered as purely inductive. By representing the consumer loads as series impedances, calculate the magnitudes of the 5th, 7th, 11th and 13th harmonic voltages at the busbar.

The system model at harmonic frequencies is as shown. From the data, the conditions at 50 Hz can be found

$$|I_A| = 380\,000/(\sqrt{3} \times 11\,000) = 19.94 \text{ A}$$
$$Z_A = 11\,000 \times (0.95 + 0.312\text{j})/(\sqrt{3} \times 19.94) = 302.6 + 99.4\text{j} \ \Omega$$
$$(L_A = 0.316 \text{ H})$$
$$|I_B| = 485\,300/(\sqrt{3} \times 11\,000) = 25.47 \text{ A}$$
$$Z_B = 11\,000 \times (0.75 + 0.661\text{j})/(\sqrt{3} \times 25.47) = 187 + 164.8\text{j} \ \Omega$$
$$(L_B = 0.525 \text{ H})$$
$$|Z_S| = 11\,000^2/(30 \times 10^6) = 4.03 \ \Omega$$
$$(L_S = 12.8 \text{ mH})$$
$$|Z_c| = 11\,000^2/247\,100 = 489.7 \ \Omega$$
$$(C = 6.5 \ \mu\text{F})$$

Busbar harmonic voltage

$$V_h = Z_{eh} I_h$$

where

Z_{eh} is the effective harmonic impedance formed by the individual harmonic impedances Z_{Ah}, Z_{Bh}, Z_{Sh} and Z_{Ch} in parallel. From above:

$$Z_{Ah} = 302.6 + 99.4n\text{j} \ \Omega \qquad\qquad Z_{Sh} = 4.03n\text{j} \ \Omega$$
$$Z_{Bh} = 187 + 164.8n\text{j} \ \Omega \qquad\qquad Z_{Ch} = -489.7\text{j}/n \ \Omega$$

From curves, the harmonic currents are:

$$I_5 = 19.8\% \text{ of } 4.2 \text{ A} = 0.832 \text{ A}$$
$$I_7 = 13.8\% \text{ of } 4.2 \text{ A} = 0.58 \text{ A}$$
$$I_{11} = 8.4\% \text{ of } 4.2 \text{ A} = 0.353 \text{ A}$$
$$I_{13} = 6.8\% \text{ of } 4.2 \text{ A} = 0.286 \text{ A}$$

Solving for the harmonic voltages gives

Harmonic	5	7	11	13
V_{hn} (V)	19.8	24.9	230	45.7

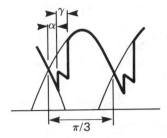

Fig. 6.5 Output voltage waveform for a six pulse, fully controlled bridge.

DC System Harmonics

The output voltage waveform of a fully-controlled converter will contain harmonic components at frequencies which are multiples of the ripple frequency. Figures 6.5 shows the DC voltage waveform for a six-pulse converter supplying a constant DC current with a firing angle of α and an overlap angle of γ. This voltage can be represented by Equations 6.9. 6.10 and 6.11.

$$v_d = V_m \cos (\omega t + \pi/6) \qquad\qquad 0 < \omega t < \alpha \qquad\qquad (6.9)$$
$$v_d = V_m [\cos (\omega t + \pi/6) + \cos (\omega t - \pi/6)]/2 \quad \alpha < \omega t < (\alpha + \gamma) \qquad (6.10)$$
$$v_d = V_m \cos (\omega t - \pi/6) \qquad\qquad (\alpha + \gamma) < \omega t < \pi/3 \qquad (6.11)$$

From these equations the RMS magnitudes of the nth harmonic component of the DC voltage waveform can be obtained in terms of the overlap angle γ, by Fourier analysis as Equation 6.12,

$$V_n = V_0 \{(n - 1)^2 \cos^2 [(n + 1)\gamma/2] + (n + 1)^2 \cos^2 [(n - 1)\gamma/2]$$
$$- 2(n - 1)(n + 1) \cos [(n + 1)\gamma/2] \cos [(n - 1)\gamma/2] \cos (2\alpha + \gamma)\}^{1/2}$$
$$1/[\sqrt{2} (n^2 - 1) \qquad\qquad (6.12)$$

where V_0 is the maximum value of mean DC voltage and n is the harmonic number

$V_0 = 3V_m/\pi$
See Equation 2.20 in Chapter 2.

With $\alpha = 0°$ and $\gamma = 0°$,

$$V_n = \sqrt{2} V_0/(n^2 - 1) \approx \sqrt{2} V_0/n^2 \qquad\qquad (6.13)$$

As α is increased the harmonic content increases. With $\alpha = 90°$ and $\gamma = 0°$,

$$V_n = \sqrt{2} V_0 n/(n^2 - 1) \approx \sqrt{2} V_0/n \qquad\qquad (6.14)$$

an increase of n times in the amplitude of the harmonic voltage. Figure 6.6 shows the relationship between harmonic voltage amplitude and overlap angle of Equation 6.12 plotted at various firing angles (α) for the 6th harmonic.

Inverter Harmonics

For the single-phase inverter with a squarewave output the voltage contains odd harmonics only, such that the nth harmonic voltage is:

$$V_n = V_1/n \qquad\qquad (6.15)$$

where V_1 is the fundamental amplitude

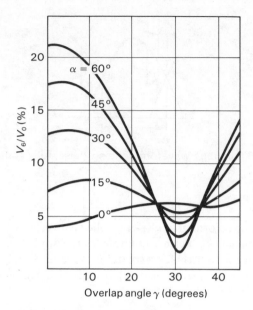

Fig. 6.6 Variation of sixth harmonic voltage content in the output of a six pulse bridge converter.

If voltage control is applied to modify the output to quasi-squarewave form then, by reference to Fig. 6.1 and Equation 6.1, the amplitudes of the individual harmonics can be expressed in terms of the amplitude of the fundamental as:

See also Equation 6.1.

$$V_n = V_1 \sin(n\psi/2)/[n \sin(\psi/2)] \tag{6.16}$$

where ψ is as shown in Fig. 6.1

The output of each phase of the basic three-phase bridge inverter discussed in Chapter 3 corresponds to that of a single-phase inverter with $\psi = 2\pi/3$. Hence the harmonic content of each phase of the AC supply can be determined by reference to Equation 6.16.

Bird, B.M. and King, K.G. (1985). *An Introduction to Power Electronics*. John Wiley.

For a pulse-width-modulated inverter the output harmonics can be controlled by the pattern of switching adopted. At any fundamental switching frequency each chop per half cycle can generally be used to eliminate one harmonic or to reduce a group of harmonic amplitudes. For r chops per half cycle one must be used to control the fundamental amplitude leaving $(r - 1)$ degrees of freedom. These may then be used to eliminate $(r - 1)$ specific low-order harmonics or to minimize the effect of a defined range of harmonics. As the total harmonic RMS voltage cannot change, the elimination of any particular harmonic will cause its contribution to this voltage to be distributed over the remaining harmonics.

In designing a PWM inverter system, a control strategy must be chosen which will achieve the desired variation of harmonic amplitude with frequency with an appropriate reduction of both harmonic torques in a motor load and overall harmonic power loss.

Worked Example 6.3   A pulse-width-modulated inverter switches the supply in the following sequence in one half cycle:

148

(a) 26.63°, on; (b) 34.2°, off; (c) 53.95°, on; (d) 66.9° off; (e) 82.61°, on; (f) 97.39°, off; (g) 113.1°, on; (h) 126.05°, off; (i) 145.8°, on; (j) 153.37°, off.

Find the amplitude of the harmonic components up to the 20th of this waveform in relation to the amplitude of the fundamental component.

The waveform contains only sine terms at odd harmonic frequencies. By applying symmetry:

$$b_n = \frac{4V_s}{\pi} \left(\int_{26.63°}^{34.2°} \sin n\theta \, d\theta + \int_{53.95°}^{66.9°} \sin n\theta \, d\theta + \int_{82.61°}^{90°} \sin n\theta \, d\theta \right)$$
$$= [\cos(26.63n) + \cos(53.95n) + \cos(82.61n) - \cos(34.2n) - \cos(66.9n)]$$

Solving,

$b_1 = 0.5; b_3 = 6.48 \times 10^{-4}; b_5 = -5.23 \times 10^{-4}; b_7 = -5.25 \times 10^{-4}$
$b_9 = = 4.45 \times 10^{-2}; b_{11} = -0.361; b_{13} = 0.361; b_{15} = 4.31 \times 10^{-2};$
$b_{17} = 1.49 \times 10^{-3}; b_{19} = 1.67 \times 10^{-2}$

Integral Cycle Control

With this type of controller the AC source frequency can no longer be used as the fundamental frequency for Fourier analysis. Consider a controller giving an ON period of N cycles, repeated every M cycles. The repetition interval is then M/f seconds and the fundamental frequency f_0 is f/M Hz. Referring to Fig. 6.7, in the interval $\omega_0 = 2\pi f_0$:

The fundamental frequency is set by the period over which the waveform repeats.

f is the frequency of the supply in hertz.

$$i_1 = I_m \sin(M\omega_0 t) \tag{6.17}$$

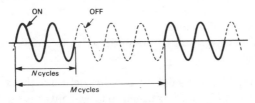

Fig. 6.7 Integral cycle control.

The waveform and period shown can be represented by a Fourier series. Therefore:

$$b_n = \frac{2}{\pi} \int_0^{N\pi/M} [I_m \sin(M\omega_0 t) \sin n\omega_0 t] \, d(\omega t)$$
$$= (-1)^N I_m 2M \sin(Nn\pi/M)/[\pi(M^2 - n^2] \tag{6.18}$$

When $n = kM$, $k = 2, 3, 4, 5$, etc. then $b_n = 0$.

Integral cycle control of this type therefore produces no harmonics of the supply frequency but generates inter-harmonic and *sub-harmonic* frequency components.

Sub-harmonics are the principle source of flicker. This is often a problem where lighting circuits, particularly using fluorescent lights, are affected. Flicker is controlled by standards such as BS5406 and IEC555.

An integral cycle controller is working from a 50 Hz supply. For the switching

Worked Example 6.4

sequence of one cycle on followed by four cycles off, find the amplitudes of the first 20 harmonics.

The sequence repeats every five cycles, hence the fundamental frequency f_1 is $50/5 = 10$ Hz.

For the case given, $N = 1$ and $M = 5$ in Equation 6.18. Substituting in this equation for $n = 1$ to $n = 20$ gives:

f_1 (10 Hz) = 0.087	f_2 (20 Hz) = 0.14
f_3 (30 Hz) = 0.189	f_4 (40 Hz) = 0.208
f_5 (50 Hz)* = 0.2	f_6 (60 Hz) = 0.17
f_7 (70 Hz) = 0.126	f_8 (80 Hz) = 0.078
f_9 (90 Hz) = 0.033	f_{10} (100 Hz)* = 0
f_{11} (110 Hz) = 0.019	f_{12} (120 Hz) = 0.025
f_{13} (130 Hz) = 0.021	f_{14} (140 Hz) = 0.011
f_{15} (150 Hz)* = 0	f_{16} (160 Hz) = 0.008
f_{17} (170 Hz) = 0.011	f_{18} (180 Hz) = 0.01
f_{19} (190 Hz) = 0.006	f_{20} (200 Hz)* = 0

Frequencies marked * are harmonics of the 50 Hz supply.

Harmonic Filters

Where harmonics present a problem on the AC system, filters can be used at the input to the converter to control their level by providing a shunt path of low impedance at the harmonic frequency. Problems in filter design include:

(a) Variation in supply (fundamental) frequency from its nominal value.
(b) Effects of ageing causing changes in filter component values and hence variation in the tuned frequency.
(c) Initial off-tuning as a result of manufacturing tolerances and the size of the tuning steps used.

The cost of providing filters is generally high in relation to the cost of the converter and their application tends to be confined to large converters or for the control of specific problems.

Tuned filters

The single tuned filter shown in Fig. 6.8 is a series RLC curcuit which is tuned to a harmonic frequency. Its impedance is given by:

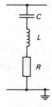

Fig. 6.8   Single tuned filter.

$$Z_f = R + j(\omega L - 1/\omega C) \tag{6.19}$$

which reduces to R at the resonance frequency f_n. The filter passband (PB) is bounded by the frequencies f_1 and f_2 at which

$$|(\omega L - 1/\omega C)| = R \tag{6.20}$$

when

$$|Z_f| = \sqrt{2}R \tag{6.21}$$

The passband is related to the quality factor (Q) by

$$Q = \omega_n|(f_2 - f_1)| \tag{6.22}$$

where $\omega_n = 2\pi f_n$

The performance of the filter is determined largely by its quality factor and the relative frequency deviation (δ), defined by Equation 6.23.

$$\omega = \omega_n(1 + \delta) \tag{6.23}$$

where ω is the actual frequency

δ may also be expressed in terms of a change in the value of L or C as

$$\delta = \frac{\Delta f}{f} + \frac{1}{2}\left(\frac{\Delta L}{L} + \frac{\Delta C}{C}\right) \tag{6.24}$$

The quality factor is given by

$$Q = \omega_n L/R = 1/\omega_n CR \tag{6.25}$$

After manipulation of Equations 6.19, 6.23 and 6.25, the impedance of the filter can be expressed by:

$$Z_f = R[1 + jQ\delta(2 + \delta)/(1 + \delta)] \tag{6.26}$$

which, if $\delta \ll 1$, can be approximated by:

$$Z_f \approx R(1 + j2\delta Q) \tag{6.27}$$

when

$$|Z_f| \approx R(1 + 4\delta^2 Q^2)^{1/2} \tag{6.28}$$

also

$$Y_f = 1/Z_f \tag{6.29}$$

The harmonic voltage at the filter is then

$$V_n = I_n/(Y_n + Y_s) \tag{6.30}$$

where Y_s is the system admittance at the point of connecting the filter

In order to estimate the maximum value of V_n likely to be encountered, the largest anticipated value of δ and the worst system admittance must be used.

A tuned filter with a Q of 30 is to be used to control the 7th harmonic content of a 50 Hz supply. The filter is constructed using a capacitor and inductor of tolerance

$f_n = \omega_n/2\pi = 1/(2\pi LC)$.

Under these conditions at the upper and lower bandwidth frequencies, Z_f has a phase angle of 45°.

ω_n is the filter tuned frequency.

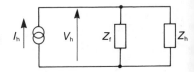

Effective impedance

$$= Z_{he} = \frac{Z_f \cdot Z_h}{Z_f + Z_h}$$

The system harmonic equivalent circuit including the filter is:

Worked Example 6.5

151

$\pm 1\%$ and $\pm 2\%$ respectively. The supply frequency can vary by ± 1 Hz. What will be the ratio between the nominal impedance of the filter and the possible worst case impedance?

From Equation 6.22

$$\delta = 0.02 + \tfrac{1}{2}(0.02 + 0.01) = 0.035$$

From Equation 6.25

$$|Z_f| = R(1 + 4 \times 0.035^2 \times 30^2)^{\frac{1}{2}} = 2.326R$$

Nominal impedance $= R$

Thus Ratio $= 2.326{:}1$

Double tuned filters

The effective impedance of the two single tuned filters of Fig. 6.9(a) about their resonance frequencies is very similar to that of the double tuned filter of Fig. 6.9(b) provided that

$$C_a = C_1 + C_2 \tag{6.31}$$

$$C_b = C_1C_2(C_1 + C_2)(L_1 + L_2)^2/(L_1C_1 - L_2C_2)^2 \tag{6.32}$$

$$L_a = \frac{L_1L_2}{L_1 + L_2} \tag{6.33}$$

$$L_b = \frac{(L_1C_1 - L_2C_2)^2}{(C_1 + C_2)^2 (L_1 + L_2)^2} \tag{6.34}$$

and

$$R_b = R_1 \left\{ \frac{a^2 (1 - b^2)}{(1 + ab^2)^2 (1 + b^2)} \right\} + R_2 \left\{ \frac{1 - b^2}{(1 + ab^2)^2 (1 + b^2)} \right\}$$
$$+ R_a \left\{ \frac{(1 - b^2)(1 - ab^2)}{(1 + ab^2)(1 + b^2)} \right\} \tag{6.35}$$

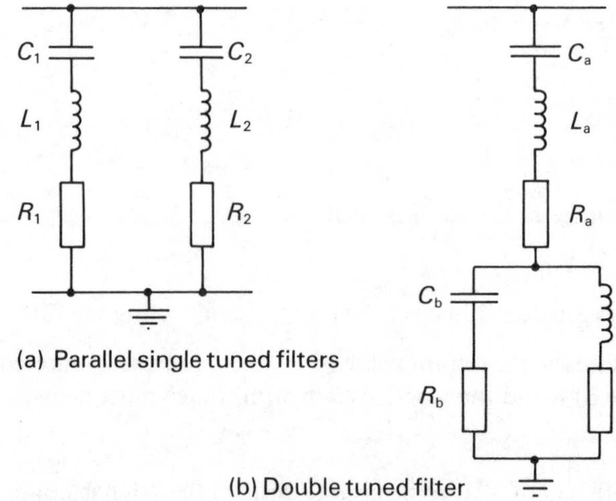

(a) Parallel single tuned filters

(b) Double tuned filter

Fig. 6.9   Double tuned filter.

where $a = C_1/C_2$ and $b = [(L_2C_2)/(L_1C_1)]^{1/2}$

The double tuned filter offers advantages in high-voltage applications as it reduces the impulse voltage rating of the inductors. Triple and quadruple tuned filters could also be produced but are difficult to adjust and are rarely used.

Automatically Tuned Filters

If the filters can be retuned to accomodate system changes this allows a higher Q filter to be produced, permitting the use of a lower rated capacitor. Tuning can be achieved by either switching capacitance or varying inductance. The control system operates by measuring the reactive power component in the filter at the harmonic frequency and then adjusts the tuning to reduce this component to as near zero as practical.

Damped filters

Various types of damped filter are shown in Fig. 6.10. Such filters are less sensitive to variations in frequency, component tolerances and temperature than tuned filters. In addition they provide a low impedance over a wide range of harmonics without the need for parallel branches and associated switching. Their disadvantages are that they need to be designed with higher fundamental VA ratings and the losses are generally higher than equivalent tuned filters.

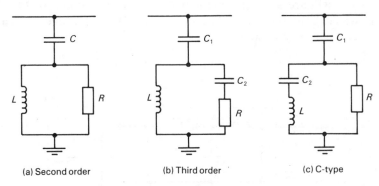

(a) Second order   (b) Third order   (c) C-type

Fig. 6.10   Damped filters.

Standards

There exist a number of national and international standards, guidelines and recommendations for the control of the harmonic levels on a power system. In each case the aim is to control the system harmonic content in such a way as to provide consumers with a waveform suited to their needs and to minimize interference with system components and communications networks while allowing for the use of distortion-producing loads. The actual form of the standard is determined by the overall requirements of the power system and is therefore a function of that system. Table 6.1 list a number of these standards.

System standards are used to control the levels of harmonic on the transmission and distribution networks. In addition to the system standards there are several appliance and equipment standards which govern the amount of distortion that can be produced by individual items of equipment.

Table 6.1   Standards for the Control of System Harmonic Content

United Kingdom	Engineering Recommendation G5/3: 1976. *Limits for Harmonics in the United Kingdom.*
Australia	Australian Standard AS2279, Parts 1 and 2: 1979. *Disturbances in Mains Supply Network.*
New Zealand	New Zealand Ministry of Energy: 1981. *Limitation of Harmonic Levels Notice.*
France	Électricité de France: 1981. *Regulations Governing the Installation of Power Converters, Taking into Account the Characteristics of the Supply Network.*

Radio-frequency Interference

The rapid transition of current that occurs when a thyristor is switched gives rise to both mains-borne noise and radiated noise in the radio-frequency range. The radiated component of radio-frequency interference (RFI) can largely be eliminated by the proper screening of the equipment and conductors. However, to control the mains-borne components some form of filtering, as shown in Fig. 6.11, will be required.

The levels of RFI are controlled in the frequency range 150 kHz to 30 MHz by standards which limit the line-to-line (symmetrical) voltage and line-to-earth (asymmetrical) voltage components.

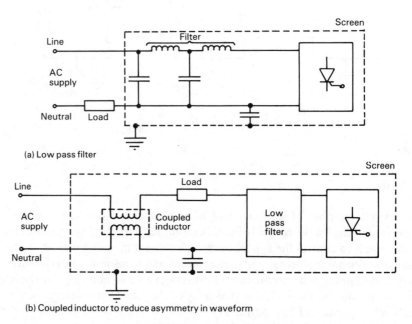

(a) Low pass filter

(b) Coupled inductor to reduce asymmetry in waveform

Fig. 6.11   RFI filtering.

Problems

6.1 Plot curves showing the variation in the harmonics, up to the 7th harmonic, with firing angle, in the supply current and load voltage of a half-controlled, single-phase rectifier supplying a constant AC current.

6.2 Repeat Problem 6.1 for the load voltage of a three-phase, half-controlled rectifier.

6.3 A three-phase fully-controlled converter operating at a firing angle of 30° with an overlap angle of 8° is drawing on r.m.s. current of 16 A from a three-phase, 11 kV, 50 Hz supply busbar. Also connected to the busbar is an effective star-connected load, each phase of which consists of a series impedance at 50 Hz of $(200 + 110j)$ Ω in parallel with a capacitive impedance at 50 Hz of $-840j$ Ω. The busbar is fed from the three-phase, 132 kV system by a 12 MVA transformer and the system fault level measured at the busbar side of the transformer is 50 MVA.

Calculate the magnitudes of the 5th, 7th, 11th and 13th harmonic currents in the 132 kV system and the corresponding harmonic voltages at the busbar.

Appendix 1 — Three-phase Systems

Phase Voltages

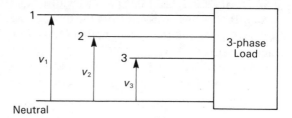

v_1, v_2 and v_3 are measured with respect to the neutral and are the *phase* voltages.

$$v_1 = V \sin(\omega t) \qquad \text{(A1.1)}$$
$$v_2 = V \sin(\omega t - 2\pi/3) \qquad \text{(A1.2)}$$
$$v_3 = V \sin(\omega t - 4\pi/3) = V \sin(\omega t + 2\pi/3) \qquad \text{(A1.3)}$$

Expressed as *phase* quantities, v_1 as reference

$$\tilde{V}_1 = V_{\text{phase}} \,\underline{|0°} \qquad \text{(A1.4)}$$
$$\tilde{V}_2 = V_{\text{phase}} \,\underline{|-120°} \qquad \text{(A1.5)}$$
$$\tilde{V}_3 = V_{\text{phase}} \,\underline{|-240°} = V_{\text{phase}} \,\underline{|120°} \qquad \text{(A1.6)}$$

where

$$V_{\text{phase}} = V/\sqrt{2}$$

and is the RMS voltage.
Also

$$V_1 + V_2 + V_3 = 0 \qquad \text{(A1.7)}$$

Line Voltages

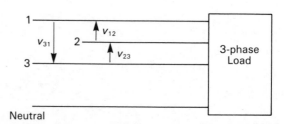

The *line* voltages are measured between pairs of lines as shown in Fig. A1.2.

$$v_{12} = v_1 - v_2 = 3V\sin(\omega t + \pi/6) \tag{A1.8}$$
$$v_{23} = v_2 - v_3 = 3V\sin(\omega t - \pi/2) \tag{A1.9}$$
$$v_{31} = v_3 - v_1 = 3V\sin(\omega t - 7\pi/6) = 3V\sin(\omega t + 5\pi/6) \tag{A1.10}$$

Expressed as *phasor* quantities, v_1 as reference

$$\tilde{V}_{12} = \tilde{V}_1 - \tilde{V}_2 = \sqrt{3}\,V_{\text{phase}}\,\underline{|30°} = V_{\text{line}}\,\underline{|30°} \tag{A1.11}$$
$$\tilde{V}_{23} = \tilde{V}_2 - \tilde{V}_3 = \sqrt{3}\,V_{\text{phase}}\,\underline{|-90°} = V_{\text{line}}\,\underline{|-90°} \tag{A1.12}$$
$$\tilde{V}_{31} = \tilde{V}_3 - \tilde{V}_1 = \sqrt{3}\,V_{\text{phase}}\,\underline{|-210°} = \sqrt{3}\,V_{\text{phase}}\,\underline{|150°} = V_{\text{line}}\,\underline{|150°} \tag{A1.13}$$

Also

$$\tilde{V}_{12} + \tilde{V}_{23} + \tilde{V}_{31} = 0 \tag{A1.14}$$

and

$$|V_{\text{line}}| = \sqrt{3}\,|V_{\text{phase}}| \tag{A1.15}$$

Appendix 2   Fourier Analysis

The Fourier series of a periodic function $x(t)$ of period T has the form

$$x(t) = a_0 + \sum_{n=1}^{\infty} \{a_n \cos(2\pi nt/T) + b_n \sin(2\pi nt/T)\} \tag{A2.1}$$

where a_0 is the mean value of the function $x(t)$, while a_n and b_n, the series coefficients are the rectangular components of the nth harmonic.

The magnitude of the nth harmonic is:

$$A_n = (a_n^2 + b_n^2)^{\frac{1}{2}} \tag{A2.2}$$

at a phase angle of

$$\phi_n = \tan^{-1}(b_n/a_n) \tag{A2.3}$$

a_0, a_n and b_n are calculated from

$$a_0 = \frac{1}{T} \int_{-T/2}^{T/2} x(t)\, dt = \frac{1}{2\pi} \int_{-\pi}^{\pi} x(\omega t)\, d(\omega t) \tag{A2.4}$$

$$a_n = \frac{2}{T} \int_{-T/2}^{T/2} x(t) \cos(2\pi nt/T)\, dt = \frac{1}{\pi} \int_{-\pi}^{\pi} x(\omega t) \cos(n\omega t)\, d(\omega t) \tag{A2.5}$$

$$b_n = \frac{2}{T} \int_{-T/2}^{T/2} x(t) \sin(2\pi nt/T)\, dt = \frac{1}{\pi} \int_{-\pi}^{\pi} x(\omega t) \sin(n\omega t)\, d(\omega t) \tag{A2.6}$$

The above may be simplified by the use of waveform symmetry.

Odd symmetry

The waveform has odd symmetry when

$$x(t) = -x(-t) \tag{A2.7}$$

in which case the a_n coefficients have a value of zero for all n and the Fourier series will contain only sine terms.

Even symmetry

The waveform has even symmetry when

$$x(t) = x(-t) \tag{A2.8}$$

in which case the b_n coefficients have a value of zero for all n and the Fourier series will contain only cosine terms.

Halfwave symmetry

The function has halfwave symmetry when

$$x(t) = -x(t + t/2) \tag{A2.9}$$

in which case the Fourier series will contain odd order harmonics only.

Reference

Arrilaga, J., Bradley, D.A. and Bodger, P.S. (1985). *Power System Harmonics*. John Wiley, U.K.

Answers to Problems

1.1 (a) 44.41 W; 36.78 A
   (b) 9.45 W; 12.7 A
   (c) 46.82 W; 35.96 A

1.2 Turn-on

t (μs)	5	10	15	20	25	30	35	40
Power (W)	840	1440	1800	1920	1800	1440	840	0

Turn-off

t (μs)	5	10	15	20	25	30	35	40	45	50	55
Power (W)	586.7	1066.7	1440	1706	1866.7	1920	1866.7	1706	1440	1066.7	586.7

1.3 1.94°C/W; 104°C

1.4 31°C

1.5 (a) $I_1 = 363$ A; $I_2 = 37$ A
   (b) $I_1 = 558$ A; $I_2 = 242$ A
   (c) $I_1 = 752.9$ A; $I_2 = 447.1$ A
   (d) $I_1 = 947.9$ A; $I_2 = 652.1$ A
   (e) $I_1 = 1142.9$ A; $I_2 = 857.1$ A
   $R = 0.445$ mΩ;
   400 A load; $I_1 = 256.8$ A; $I_2 = 143.2$ A
   2000 A load; $I_1 = 1049.8$ A; $I_2 = 950.2$ A

1.6 $V_1 = 2432$ V; $V_2 = 2288$ V; $V_3 = 2480$ V
   $I_1 = 81.1$ A; $I_2 = 76.27$ A, $I_3 = 82.67$ A

2.1 For a resistive load current is in phase with voltage a the conduction angle is $(180 - \alpha)°$
   $\alpha = 30°$; $I_{mean} = 6.16$ A; $I_{max} = 20.74$ A; $I_{RMS} = 10.22$ A
   $\alpha = 60°$; $I_{mean} = 4.95$ A; $I_{max} = 20.74$ A; $I_{RMS} = 10.07$ A
   Firing angle = 20° 39′

2.2 $\alpha = 0°$; Power = 11.2 kW
   $\alpha = 75°$; Power = 2.9 kW

2.3 The waveform will be as Fig. 2.3(b)

2.4 Turn-on, overlap = 0.9°
   Turn-off, overlap = 9.5°

2.5 Primary rating = 23.8 kW; Secondary rating = 33.7 kW

2.6 $\alpha = 63°$ 10′; $I_{RMS} = 34.64$ A; Power = 24 W
   $\alpha = 58°$ 23′

2.7 Thyristor rating, Series = 288.67 A; Parallel = 144.33 A
   Transformer rating = 18.5 MW

2.8 (a) $2\sqrt{2} \cos \alpha/\pi$ (b) Power factor = $\sqrt{2}(1 + \cos \alpha)/\{\pi(\pi - \alpha)\}^{1/2}$

2.9 Voltage = 506.6 V; $\gamma = 8°$ 17′; $\delta = 21°$ 43′

2.10 $I = 67.53$ A

3.1 (a) 189.3 W; (b) 134.4 W

3.2 (a) $V = 55$ V; $I = 11$ A

    (b) $V = 91.67$ V; $I = 18.33$ A

    (c) $V = 27.5$ V; $I = 5.5$ A

3.3 $L = 0.654$ mH; $C = 14.1$ μF

3.4 (a) 5829 W (b) 3352 W

3.5 $L = 12.5$H, $C = 1.8$ μF

3.6 $V = 998$ V (line)

    Peak current = 101.8 A

    Tyristor RMS current = 58.8 A

    Load power = 29.4 kW; Input power factor = 0.41

4.1 237 rpm

4.2 (i) 14.86 Nm

    (ii) 18.28°, 22.98 Nm

4.3 13.08 Nm

4.4 See notes on pages 102 and 103

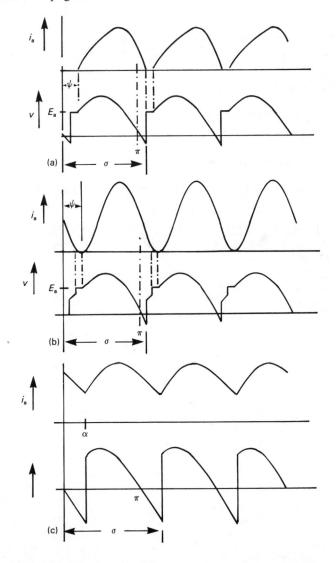

4.5 (a) 1267 rpm; (b) 1599 rpm; (c) 107 Nm; (d) 56.7 Nm
4.6 (iv) 107.7 V (v) 41.48 V
4.7 72.08°

5.1 $I_{RMS} = 1804$ A; Peak reverse voltage = 167.6 kV
5.2 Rating (RMS) = 33.39 A
@ 16 kW $\alpha = 74.49°$
@ 8 kW $\alpha = 105.29°$
Thyristor rating (RMS) = 23.61 A
5.3 (a) 3441 W; (b) 1370 W; (c) 177.2 W
5.4 $V_L = V_{max} \left(\dfrac{1}{\pi} \left[\dfrac{\pi}{2} - \dfrac{5\alpha}{18} + \dfrac{10}{18} \sin 2\alpha \right] \right)^{\frac{1}{2}}$
5.5 0.559 mH

6.1 Voltage
$a_n = 0$ for n odd
$= \dfrac{V_m}{\pi} \left[\dfrac{2}{1 - n^2} + \dfrac{\cos [(1 + n)\alpha]}{1 + n} + \dfrac{\cos [(1 - n)\alpha]}{1 - n} \right]$ n even
$b_n = 0$ for n odd
$= \dfrac{V_m}{\pi} \left[\dfrac{\sin [(1 + n)\alpha]}{1 + n} - \dfrac{\sin [(1 - n)\alpha]}{1 - n} \right]$ n even
Current
$a_n = 0$ for n even
$= -\dfrac{2}{n\pi} \sin (n\alpha)$ for n odd
$b_n = 0$ for n even
$= \dfrac{2}{n\pi} (1 + \cos (n\alpha))$ for n odd
6.2 $a_n = \dfrac{3}{2\pi} \left[\dfrac{\sin [(3n + 1)\alpha]}{3n + 1} + \dfrac{\sin [(1 - 3n)\alpha]}{1 - 3n} - \dfrac{\sqrt{3} \cos (n\pi)}{1 - 9n^2} \right]$
$b_n = \dfrac{3}{2\pi} \left[\dfrac{\cos [(1 + 3n)\alpha]}{1 + 3n} + \dfrac{\cos [(1 - 3n)\alpha]}{1 - 3n} - \dfrac{\cos (n\pi)}{1 - 9n^2} \right]$
6.3 $I_5 = 0.277$ A
$I_7 = 0.22$ A
$I_{11} = 0.238$ A
$I_{13} = 0.459$ A

Index